Nursing Research in Action

Developing Basic Skills

Second Edition

Philip Burnard
Director of Postgraduate Nursing Studies
University of Wales College of Medicine
Cardiff

and

Paul Morrison
Senior Lecturer
University of Wales College of Medicine
Cardiff

MACMILLAN

First edition 1990
Reprinted three times
Second edition 1994

Published by
MACMILLAN PRESS LTD
Houndmills, Basingstoke, Hampshire RG21 2XS
and London
Companies and representatives
throughout the world

ISBN 0–333–60876–3

A catalogue record for this book is available
from the British Library.

10 9   8   7   6   5   4   3
03 02 01 00 99 98 97 96

Printed in Great Britain by
Antony Rowe Ltd, Chippenham

To Sally, Aaron and Rebecca
and
for Franziska, Sarah and Maeve

Acknowledgements

The authors would like to thank Bunny le Roux, Principal Lecturer, Department of Applied Statistics and Operational Research, Sheffield Hallam University for permission to reproduce the statistical exercise in Chapter 8; and the Science and Engineering Research Council for permission to adapt material from *An Approach to Good Supervisory Practice* (1983).

Every effort has been made to trace all the copyright holders, but if any have been inadvertently overlooked the publishers will be pleased to make the necessary arrangement at the first opportunity.

Contents

About the Authors

Philip Burnard

Philip is Director of Postgraduate Nursing Studies at the University of Wales College of Medicine and Honorary Lecturer in Nursing at the Hogeschool Midden Nederland. He has carried out a variety of research projects including ones into experiential learning, AIDS counselling, interpersonal skills and forensic psychiatric nursing. Author of a variety of books about nursing and health care issues, he is a frequent contributor to the nursing press.

Paul Morrison

Paul is a Senior Lecturer at the University of Wales College of Medicine, where he teaches the psychology component of the Bachelor of Nursing course. He is a chartered psychologist and an Associate Fellow of the British Psychological Society. Author of a number of books, his research interests include the provision of psychological care in health care settings, management of disturbed behaviour in psychiatric care, and assessment of interpersonal communication skills.

Preface

Research is a means of understanding, assessing and evaluating what we do as nurses. It can help us to plan for the future. It can be exciting and satisfying. It can also be hard work. If you are just beginning to study research this book will help you to think ahead and to anticipate the stages of the research process. It will also help you to develop certain basic research skills that are common to all research. Whilst research is never a clear-cut and tidy process, one alternative to being overwhelmed by the task and giving up is to develop structure. In this book we develop a structured approach to research.

The book aims to make research into nursing possible for those who are just setting out in the field. It offers a series of achievable exercises in all the phases of the research process. As you do the exercises you will begin to follow the process of how to do research yourself, or to develop an understanding of what other researchers have done. We suggest that after you have finished working through this book, you do a small piece of research yourself. However, we do not suggest that you do it alone. As we noted above, research is often hard work and uses a whole range of skills. It is not something to be rushed into.

It is not our intention that this book should stand alone. It is a book that can be used as a guide alongside other texts on research. It should also be used in conjunction with a tutor and with other nursing colleagues.

We are both nurses and both teach research methods. Driven by the idea that there is no better way to learn to do something than by doing it, we have undertaken a number of research projects both large-scale and small. We have also supervised the research projects of students. In the process we have learned some things about doing research. We have learned, for instance, that there is no one 'right' way to do research. We have also learned that one of the best ways to learn research is to do it. We hope that this book will allow you to sample various aspects of the research process as a means of building up a range of research skills and confidence in evaluating research which you might use.

The book may be used in a variety of ways:

- It may be used on its own as a learning package. A nurse working through the book on his/her own can do the various exercises and follow up the various approaches through reference to the various books and articles recommended throughout the text. S(he) may also do further reading via the extended recommended reading list at the back of the book. The compendium of research resources, also at the back of the book, will be a further aid.
- The book may also be used as part of a student-centred learning programme. Nurse educators are realising, increasingly, that people learn at different speeds and that their learning needs vary. Thus, the book can be tailored to suit the varying needs of the people using it. For some, it will help to work right through the book as an introduction to research methods. For others, it will be more appropriate to select certain chapters relating to specific skills.
- It may be used as a programme of guided reading. The book unfolds logically to cover all the stages of the research process. As it does this, a wide and varied range of references is offered. Readers are given the opportunity to sample different sorts of research. Thus the book can be a rich source of reference for the person who wishes to become familiar with a broad view of the research literature. Examples of research projects are drawn not only from nursing but from the whole range of social sciences. We feel that it is important that nurses sample and explore all sorts of approaches to doing research.
- The book may be used as a resource. Many of the passages can serve as the means by which ideas are sparked off or the next stage of a research project is planned. The references offered throughout the book and in the bibliography will also be useful in gaining new leads and developing thoughts and plans.
- Experiential learning, or learning directly through personal experience, is also a growing trend in nurse education. The book is not only theoretical in nature. It invites the reader to complete a range of exercises to reinforce learning. Thus, used in a group context and with group reflection after the completion of each exercise, the book can be used as an aid to facilitating experiential learning. If the book is used in this way, it is recommended that the following issues are born in mind:
- The tutor or facilitator should appreciate that each student will tend to find different results at the end of each exercise. It is useful if the tutor does not try to force a particular point of view on the group but allows for these differences of perception.
- Plenty of time should be allowed for the completion of the exercises and about an hour should be allowed afterwards for discussion or 'processing' of the activity.

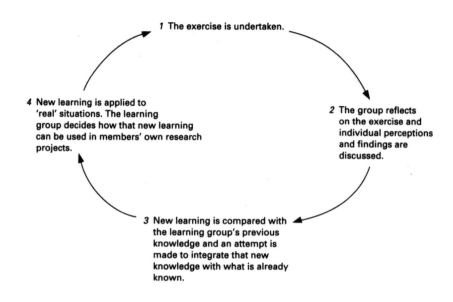

1 The exercise is undertaken.

2 The group reflects on the exercise and individual perceptions and findings are discussed.

3 New learning is compared with the learning group's previous knowledge and an attempt is made to integrate that new knowledge with what is already known.

4 New learning is applied to 'real' situations. The learning group decides how that new learning can be used in members' own research projects.

An experiential learning cycle applied to the exercises in this book

- It is helpful if the tutor reads through a particular exercise that is being used and makes sure that all learners have access to the various research reports and other references that are cited in the text. If nurses are to plan and carry out research projects it is essential that they have easy access to a well-stocked library. As we noted earlier, the references quoted in this book are drawn from a wide variety of sources within the social and behavioural sciences. Whilst they are all obtainable via the inter-library loan system, it is clearly more helpful to learners if they are more readily available.
- It is useful if the experiential learning cycle shown above is used in order to make full use of the exercises.

The book offers an exploratory approach to most aspects of the research cycle. Both quantitative and qualitative methods of doing research are addressed as are a variety of ways of collecting and analysing data. The reader is encouraged to draw up a research proposal, identify proposed data collection methods and methods of analysis, and is then directed towards writing up the project. A series of 'information sections' is offered throughout the text to illuminate certain aspects of the topics under discussion. At the end of the book, as we have already noted, there is a compendium containing further information on all sorts of aspects of the research process. Overall, the book should serve as a practical introduction to the business of doing research in nursing.

We have been unable to find a satisfactory solution to the problem of non-sexist language. Using 'they' as both singular and plural was considered but deemed to be clumsy. In the end, we settled for the nurse as 'she', though we wish to acknowledge that the reader may just as easily read 'he' in its place. The issue of how to write clear and unambiguous non-sexist prose remains a challenge both for the writer generally and for the person who is reporting research.

More than anything else, we hope that the book will make you *think* about the issues involved in doing research – whether or not you do your *own* research.

Cardiff, 1994   PHILIP BURNARD
                                                                                PAUL MORRISON

1

An Overview of the Research Process

Aims of this Chapter

• To identify definitions of research;
• To identify examples of different sorts of research;
• To outline the stages of the research process;
• To help you plan your research project in a structured and methodical way.

Introduction

Research has been defined in various ways. In this chapter you will be exploring some of those definitions. What is more important, however, is that almost all research goes through certain stages. If you can develop the skill of breaking down your project into manageable chunks you will find it that much easier to control and to do. The first part of the chapter invites you to think about what research is; the second part offers you a format for identifying the stages that go to make up the research process. If you begin with structure, your task will be easier and your thinking clearer.

The point of all this should be to enable you to be able to *read* research reports and make more sense of them. Also, you should be able to *apply* what you read to your own working environment and to the clinical situation. In addition, you should be able to use this level of understanding to evaluate, critically, other people's research reports and evaluate their relevance (or lack of it) to the nursing environment. In the words of the late social psychologist and researcher, Kurt Lewin: 'Research that produces nothing but books will not suffice' (Lewin, 1946).

What You Need to Read

This should include the following:

Bell, J. (1987) *Doing Your Research Project: A Guide For First-Time Researchers in Education and Social Science*, Oxford University Press, Oxford.
Cormack, D.F.S. (ed.) (1991) *The Research Process in Nursing*, 2nd edn, Blackwell, Oxford, chs 1 and 2.
Sommer, B. and Sommer, R. (1991) *A Practical Guide To Behavioural Research: Tools and Techniques*, 3rd edn, Oxford University Press, Oxford.

1.1 Definitions of Research

By the end of this section you will have discovered:

• How to define research;
• The meanings or usage of certain words.

Some Definitions of Research

Research has been defined as:

> *careful search or enquiry after or for or into; endeavour to discover new or collate old facts etc by scientific study of a subject, course of critical investigation* (*Concise Oxford Dictionary*, 7th edn, Oxford University Press, Oxford, 1982)

Here are some more definitions:

> *Research is a scientific process of inquiry and/or experimentation that involves purposeful, systematic, and rigorous collection of data. Analysis and interpretation of the data are then made in order to gain new knowledge or add to existing knowledge. Research has the ultimate aim of developing an organised body of scientific knowledge.* (Dempsey, P.A. and Dempsey, A.P. 1986, *The Research Process in Nursing*, Boston, MA: Jones & Bartlett)

> *Research is done to find out. What is happening? How does it work? Which produces better results? Which statement is true? When we want to know something and we are not satisfied with the word of authorities,*

2

we do research. (Dixon, B.R., Bouma and Atkinson, G.B.J. 1987, *A Handbook of Social Science Research*, Oxford University Press, Oxford)

Research is . . . not a luxury for the academic, but a tool for developing the quality of nursing decisions, prescriptions and actions. Whether as clinicians, educators, managers or researchers we have a research responsibility: neglect of that responsibility could be classed as, professional negligence. (McFarlane, J. 1984, *Research Process in Nursing – the Future*, in D.F.S. Cormack (ed.). *The Research Process in Nursing*, Oxford)

Empirical *research involves the measurement of observable events – for example, the effect of a particular drug on a reaction time, people's responses to questionnaires, of individual characteristics measured by a personality inventory. Empirical refers to information that is sense-based – what we directly see, hear, touch, smell or taste. It is demonstrable: that is, it can be shown to other people. Subjective qualities such as feelings and beliefs become empirical when expressed by means of attitude scales, interviews, ratings, or other some other measurement procedures.* (Sommer, B. and Sommer, R. 1991, *A Practical Guide to Behavioural Research: Tools and Techniques*, 3rd edn, Oxford University Press, Oxford)

*Scientific work depends on a mixture of boldly innovative thought and the careful marshalling of evidence to support or disconfirm hypotheses or theories. Information and insights accumulated through scientific and debate are always to some degree **tentative** – open to being revised or even completely discarded, in the light of new evidence or arguments.* (Giddens, A. 1989, *Sociology*, Polity Press, Cambridge)

Exercise 1.1

Aim of the exercise: To explore some definitions of research.

Planning stage: You can do this exercise on your own or in the company of a small group of colleagues, friends or students. Allow yourself plenty of time to complete the exercise and make notes of what you do, as you go. If you work with friends or colleagues, decide whether you will all carry out similar tasks or you will divide up the work between you.

Equipment / resources required: Notebook, pen and access to a nursing library.

What to do: Read the above definitions and consider the following questions

- In what way do these definitions disagree or agree with each other?
- What is meant by the word 'scientific' in any of the definitions?
- Can you be scientific about people?
- Which definition do you prefer and why?
- Does the dictionary definition seem any different to the others? If so, what are the problems of using a dictionary to define words with specific meanings in a particular discipline?

Read through the following research reports and then consider in what ways those pieces of research support the definitions offered above. If they do not, in what ways are the above definitions inadequate, if these reports are still to be called research?

Firth, H., McIntee, J., McKeown and Britton, P. (1986) 'Interpersonal support amongst nurses at work', *Journal of Advanced Nursing*, **11**, 273–82.

Haase, J.E. (1987) 'Components of courage in chronically ill adolescents: A phenomenological study', *Advances in Nursing Science*, **9** (2) 64–80.

Jeffery, R. (1979) 'Normal rubbish: deviant patients in casualty departments', *Sociology of Health and Illness*, **1** (1) 90–107.

Evaluation: Discuss your conclusions with colleagues and with a tutor. Can research be defined easily? What are the problems with definition in this field? Have your views about research changed as a result of reading research reports?

As another level of evaluation, it is useful, before you finish the activity, to note down:

(a) what you learned from doing the activity,
(b) how you will use what you learned,
(c) how what you have learned relates to what you have read, and
(d) what you need to learn next.

1.2 Examples of Nursing Research

By the end of this section you will have discovered:

- What types of research have been done in nursing;
- The bridges that can be formed between nursing and other disciplines;
- The wide range of issues that have been addressed by nursing researchers.

Where do you Find Research Reports?

Research is written up in a variety of books, articles and papers. The following list offers some sources of research material:

- Books
- Magazines and journals such as:
  Nursing Times (Short Reports and Occasional Papers sections)
  Journal of Advanced Nursing
  Nurse Education Today
  Nursing, the add-on journal,
  International Journal of Nursing Studies
  Also: a wide range of North American journals, available through your library.
- Newspapers
- University and college theses and dissertations (these are often available from university and college libraries on microfiche)
- Authors and researchers
- Remember that the inter-library loan system, available through most libraries, can arrange for you to see copies of research reports that are not available to you locally. Ask your librarian how this system works and how you can use it.
- CD-ROM. CD-ROM stands for 'Compact Disk: Read Only Memory'. Your library is likely to have a computer which can search special compact disks that contain huge amounts of details about nursing references and research reports. These disks often offer an *abstract* for each report: a short summary of the research aims, the research methods used and the findings of the study.

Further Reading

Akinsanya, J. (1984) 'Learning about nursing research', *Nursing Times*, **80** (16) 59–61.
Clamp, C.G.L. (1991) *Resources for Nursing Research: an annotated bibliography*, Library Association Publishing, London.
Smith, J.P. (1983) 'Steinberg Collection of Nursing Research', *Journal of Advanced Nursing*, **8** (5) 357.

Exercise 1.2

Aim of the exercise: To explore the range of research that has been done in nursing.

Planning stage: You can do this exercise on your own or in the company of a small group of colleagues, friends or students. Allow yourself plenty of time to complete the exercise and make notes of what you do, as you go. If you work with friends or colleagues, decide whether you will all carry out similar tasks or you will divide up the work between you.

Equipment / resources required: Notebook, pen and access to a nursing library.

What to do: Read a selection of chapters from the following books to discover some of the types of research that have been done in this field:

Brooking, J. (ed.) (1986) *Psychiatric Nursing Research*, Wiley, Chichester.
Clark, J.M. and Hockey, L. (1979) *Research for Nursing: A Guide for the Enquiring Nurse*, HM & M, Aylesbury.
Fielding, P. (ed.) (1987) *Research in Geriatric Nursing*, Wiley, Chichester.
While, A. (ed.) (1986) *Research in Preventive Community Nursing Care*, Wiley, Chichester.

Read the section below on 'Types of Nursing Research' to consider the range of approaches to nursing research.

Go to the librarian in your nursing library and ask to see a copy of: the *Journal of Advanced Nursing*. Look through this and make a note of some of the research studies that may relate to your own field of interest. Then note down one or two titles of research projects that are very different to your own areas of interest. Try to get copies of these reports and read them. Consider the following points:

• In what way do the various research reports differ from each other?
• To what extent are the reports related to clinical nursing?
• Were the reports easy to read? Were there difficulties with any of the following:
the terminology used?

reading tables and statistical reports?
the author's style of writing?
- What sort of structure did the reports have? Were they clearly laid out with a series of headings and sub-headings?

Evaluation: Discuss your findings with colleagues and with your tutor. Try to discover if there is a standard format for the layout of research reports. Consider, too, the wide range of:

- nursing research topics;
- approaches to research;
- ways of doing research;
- readability in nursing research reports. Remember: anyone who has anything important to say will not risk being misunderstood. Has this been true in your experience?

As another level of evaluation, it is useful, before you finish the activity, to note down:

(a) what you learned from doing the activity,
(b) how you will use what you learned,
(c) how what you have learned relates to what you have read, and
(d) what you need to learn next.

Types of Nursing Research

Some research projects are general and broad in approach: they study the broad canvas of nursing. Others look at a particular aspect of nursing, for example medical nursing. Others consider one topic in nursing, e.g. pain. Others, still, look only at one specific case or situation. In the diagram below, you can see the progression from the general to the specific. What will your project be: 'broad' in nature or in-depth and very specific?

Nursing in general: ....

Types of nursing: medical, surgical, psychiatric, etc.

Specific topics: pain, pressure sores ....

Single cases or situations: ....

7

Another way of considering types of research is to think about the theoretical framework adopted by the researcher. For example, some researchers study their topic from a psychological point of view, some from a sociological standpoint and others from a biological position. Others, of course, combine various theoretical approaches. In recent years, the nursing profession has begun to develop its own body of theories and models. Research is being done to clarify and validate that theoretical base. Below are some examples of nursing research reports which illustrate a particular theoretical position:

A psychological study: Davis, B.D. (1983) 'A repertory grid study of formal and informal aspects of student nurse training', unpublished PhD thesis, University of London.

A sociological study: Towell, D. (1975) *Understanding Psychiatric Nursing: A sociological study of modern psychiatric practice*, RCN, London.

A biological study: Hart, J.A. (1985) 'The urethral catheter – A review of its implication in urinary-tract infection', *International Journal of Nursing Studies*, **22** (1) 57–70.

A nursing study: Haggerty, L. (1987) 'An analysis of senior US nursing students immediate responses to distressed patients', *Nursing Times*, **23** (83) 57.

A social psychology study: Morrison, P. (1992) *Professional Caring in Practice: A psychological analysis*, Avebury, Aldershot.

A nursing education study: Burnard, P. (1991) *Experiential Learning in Action*, Avebury, Aldershot.

1.3 Stages of the Research Process

By the end of this section you will have discovered:

- How to divide up the task of doing research into manageable chunks.
- How to think systematically about your research.
- How most research, irrespective of the approach that is taken, is *structured*.

Exercise 1.3

Aim of the exercise: To identify the stages of the research process.

Planning stage: You can do this exercise on your own or in the company of a small group of colleagues, friends or students. Allow yourself plenty of time to complete the exercise and make notes of what you do, as you go. If you work with friends or colleagues, decide whether you will all carry out similar tasks or you will divide up the work between you.

Equipment / resources required: Notebook, pen and access to a nursing library.

What to do: Find one nursing research report from each of the following journals. Note, when you find them, differences in style, content, layout and readability in each of the journals:

• *Nurse Education Today*
• *Journal of Advanced Nursing*
• *British Journal of Nursing*
• *Nursing Research*
• *British Journal of Nursing*
• *Journal of Clinical Nursing*
• *Issues in Mental Health Nursing*.

All of these journals use headings and sub-headings in the lay-out of their research reports and articles.

Jot down the heading used in a nursing research report from each of the above journals and notice to what degree there are similarities and differences between the sorts of headings and sub-headings used. Out of this information, try to devise a system of stages that may help to guide you through the process of doing research. Then read the guidelines laid out in the section below. To what degree do your headings coincide with ours?

Evaluation: Notice the similarity between the headings used in a written report and the stages of the research process. You can use the headings that you have derived or the headings in our information box for two purposes:

• to guide you in your planning
• to help you organise the writing up of your project.

As another level of evaluation, it is useful, before you finish the activity, to note down:

(a) what you learned from doing the activity,
(b) how you will use what you learned

(c) how what you have learned relates to what you have read, and
(d) what you need to learn next.

Stages in the Research Process

One of the first tasks the researcher has to consider is the *structure* of his or
her research work. In order to facilitate this, it is useful to write out a
research proposal. The details of such a proposal are discussed later in this
book. At the moment, it is important to focus on the broad stages of the
research process and these can be enumerated as follows:

1. Deciding on the research question;
2. Locating and searching relevant literature;
3. Planning the project and preparing a proposal;
4. Considering ethical issues and getting permission to do the research.
5. Negotiating access to the research site;
6. Selecting an appropriate method;
7. Collecting and storing data;
8. Analysising and interpreting data;
9. Drawing conclusions and making recommendations;
10. Writing up and presenting the findings.

This is *one* way of planning your research. You may find other outlines.
The important thing is that you *plan*. Research is never a tidy process. You
will often find that the stages in the research process overlap in various
ways and that you will return to certain stages again and again. Despite
this, it is still important to have a very clear initial plan that can serve as a
template for your work.

Further Reading

Couchman, W. and Dawson, D. (1990) *Nursing and Health-Care Research
  – A Practical Guide: The use and application of research for nurses and
  other health care Professionals*, Scutari, London.
Gilbert, N. (ed.) (1993) *Researching Social Life*, Sage, London.
Hammersley, M. (ed.) (1993) *Social Research: Philosophy, Politics and
  Practice*, Sage, London.
Leino-Kilpi, H. and Tuomaala, U. (1989) 'Research ethics and nursing sci-
  ence: an empirical example', *Journal of Advanced Nursing*, **14**, 415–58.
Sarter, B. (ed.) (1988) *Paths to Knowledge: Innovative Research Methods
  for Nursing*, National League for Nursing, New York.

1.4 Planning your Research Project

By the end of this section you will have discovered:

• How to bring structure to your own project and how to plan your work;
• How most other researchers have always *structured* their work;
• How research is reported by reference to this structure.

Exercise 1.4

Aim of the exercise: To explore aspects of your own research project

Planning stage: This exercise should be carried out on your own. Allow yourself plenty of time to complete the exercise and make notes of what you do, as you go.

Equipment / resources required: Notebook, pen and access to a nursing library.

What to do: Make notes about your own research topic under the following headings:

1. Deciding on the Research Question
• What do you want to find out?
• Can you write *one sentence* that sums up what you want to do?

This stage of your work is critical. If you can clarify exactly what it is that you want to research, then the other processes that follow will be that much easier. It is worth investing considerable time in undertaking the clarification of your research question. Discuss this at some length with both your tutors and with other people who have had research experience. As you read more and refer to other sources of literature you may want to refine, further, your research question.

2. Locating and Searching Relevant Literature
• Where will you go to find relevant literature?
• Do you know how to use bibliographies and indexes at your library?
• Are you familiar with the inter-library loan system?

3. Planning the Project and Preparing a Proposal
- Are there specific proposal guidelines and forms issued by your school of nursing, college or local authority?
- Have you got someone to oversee your project: a supervisor?
- Have you seen other people's proposals? If not, have a look at one soon.

4. Considering Ethical Issues and Getting Permission to do the Research
- Will you be talking to patients? If so, you will probably be required to submit your proposal to an ethics committee. The issue of whether or not a research proposal should be subject to the approval of an ethics committee varies from area to area. You need to check with your own health authority or department whether or not your project will require ethical approval. This is a critical aspect of your work. You cannot proceed without ethical clearance if your area or department insist upon it.
- Could anything in your project upset the people you are interviewing or talking to? If so, is it appropriate to ask such questions? If you or the person supervising your project is in any doubt about the sensitive nature of your questions, make sure that you are taking steps to develop skills in handling sensitive responses. Otherwise, leave out any questions that could be upsetting.
- Do you know how to make a submission to your ethics committee?

5. Negotiating Access to the Research Site
- Whom do you approach to get permission to the people you want to talk to in your research? It is usual to adopt a 'top down' approach and ask the most senior person first. You MUST ask permission to interview or talk to people. You cannot assume that no one will mind if you don't bother.

6. Selecting an Appropriate Method
- What methods have been used in this field before?
- Have they been used successfully?
- Is it time for a fresh approach?
- What other approaches are available?

7. Collecting and Storing Data
- What practical considerations do you need to make with regard to collecting data? Consider, for example, the following issues:

allocation of time;

finding a place to talk to people;

expenses to cover postage, travel, typewriting/word processing;

facilities for storing data: files, paper, computer software.

8. Analysising and Interpreting Data

- Are you familiar with *how* to analyse data? This will be discussed in a later chapter but you must have decided how to analyse data before you begin to collect it.

9. Drawing Conclusions and Making Recommendations

- What sort of conclusions do you anticipate drawing? If you can answer this too readily, then you are not remaining open-minded. You are tending to pre-judge the outcome of your research.
- Who will be interested in your research? For what audience will you be writing?

10. Writing Up and Presenting the Findings

- Can you type and/or use a word processor?
- Have you got access to these things?
- If not, can you afford to have your work typed by someone else?
- Will you need to send copies of your report to other people?
- If so, is there a standard format for such a report?

Evaluation: Talk these issues through with colleagues and with your tutor. Note the learning needs that may have arisen as a result of doing this exercise and keep a note of them. The following chapters will help you to become proficient in undertaking the tasks alluded to in the above questions.

At a later stage in your work, you may want to return and do this exercise again. Your needs, wants and skills will change as you get on with doing your research.

As another level of evaluation, it is useful, before you finish the activity, to note down:

(a) what you learned from doing the activity,

(b) how you will use what you learned,

(c) how what you have learned relates to what you have read, and

(d) what you need to learn next.

Conclusion

Planning and structuring your project before you start to collect data will pay huge dividends and is a necessity. The more you are able to organise your work, the more clear you will be about the tasks you have to do. It is helpful to sit down with a large pad of paper and make a series of headings and sub-headings, thus dividing up your project into smaller and smaller tasks. This process (which is sometimes known as 'outlining') can also be done on a personal computer or word processor.

It is very hard to draw up a plan of research, and usually you will have to do a variety of *drafts*: not many people get it right first time. The plan must also be *realistic*. It is easy to think of the sort of project you would *like* to do, but often it is a question of what you *can* do. Many initial plans are overambitious. Work closely with a supervisor who has research experience and be guided by her or him.

The great advantage of planning your work properly in advance is that such planning nearly always leads to a much better outcome. Your research report will benefit from the planning that you put into place at the beginning of your study.

Learning Check

If You are Working on Your Own

Read through the notes that you have kept whilst completing the exercises in this chapter and consider the following questions:

- What new knowledge have I gained?
- What new skills have I developed?
- How has my thinking about research changed?
- What do I need to do now?

Check that you have made reference cards for any new references that you have found whilst working on the exercises in this chapter.

If You are Working in a Small Group

Pair off and nominate one of you as A and one of you as B. For five minutes, A talks to B about what she has learned and B listens. This should *not* be a conversation: B's only role is to listen. After five minutes, roles are reversed and B talks to A about what she has learned and A listens. After the second five minutes, re-form into a group and discuss the experience.

If You are a Tutor and/or Facilitator

- Use the above pairs exercise with the group you are working with.
- Hold two 'rounds' in which each person in turn says *(a)* what she liked least about doing the activities and *(b)* what she liked most about doing the activities

2

Planning Your Research Project

Aims of this Chapter

- To help clarify research problems and questions;
- To demonstrate how to write a research proposal;
- To help identify constraints in the research process.

Introduction

In this chapter we explore the process of planning the research project. In the first chapter we talked about the research proposal: your statement of intent with regard to your research. In this chapter we show you how to write one. Some of the information you need to complete a research proposal is covered in later chapters of this book. We suggest that you undertake the exercises here, now: later, and in the light of your new knowledge, you should return to this chapter and be prepared to modify your proposal.

What You Need to Read for This Chapter

Darling, V.H. and Rogers, J. (1986) *Research for Practising Nursing*, Macmillan, Basingstoke. Dempsey, P.A. and Dempsey A.D. (1986) *The Research Process in Nursing*, 2nd edn, Jones and Bartlett, Boston, MA, ch. 3.

Dixon, B.R., Buma, G.D. and Atkinson, G.B.J. (1987) *A Handbook of Social Science Research*, Oxford University Press, Oxford, ch. 3.

Herbert, M. (1990) *Planning a Research Project: A Guide for Practitioners and Trainees in the Helping Professions*, Caswell Educational, London.

Leedy, P.D. (1985) *Practical Research: Planning and Design*, 3rd edn, Macmillan, New York, chs 3, 5 and 6.

Vanetzian, E. (1987) 'Using PERT to keep a nursing research project humming', *Nursing Research*, **36** (6) 388–92.

2.1 Clarifying Research Problems and Questions

By the end of this section you will have discovered:

- How to be clear about what your research is about.
- How other people have clarified their research problems
- How important all this is in reading and evaluating research reports.

Exercise 2.1

Aim of the exercise: To identify a clear and specific research problem or question.

Planning stage: You can do this exercise on your own or in the company of a small group of colleagues, friends or students. Allow yourself plenty of time to complete the exercise and make notes of what you do, as you go. If you work with friends or colleagues, decide whether you will all carry out similar tasks or divide up the work between you.

Equipment / resources required: Notebook, pen and access to a nursing library.

What to do: For this exercise, you will be encouraged to use the process known as 'brainstorming'. It is a technique that will be useful in a variety of ways throughout your research work. The section headed 'Brainstorming' on page 19 spells out the stages in the process. Read it now.
Using the brainstorming technique, take a large sheet of paper and brainstorm all the sorts of issues that you are interested in as possible fields or aspects of research. A typical list may (or may not) look like this:

- pressure sores
- stress in nurses,
- stress in myself
- skill mixes
- interpersonal skills
- counselling skills
- care of the dying
- nursing models: do they work?
- what are nursing models?

17

Notice, as the list above has developed, questions have begun to form. This is the beginning of the process of clarification of a possible research problem or question. Note that the last two items in the above list begin to narrow in focus. You will find it helpful to be as specific as you can when you come to framing your research question. We suggest that you work with your brainstorming and prioritisation until you can frame your research problem or question in one sentence.

Some negative and positive examples of research questions are offered below: some of them will lead to systematic and logical enquiry (the positive ones), the others will need further clarification. Look through the list and mark which ones you see as being positive and which ones you see as negative. When you have completed this task, go back to your own work and further refine the question or problem until you are sure that the statement is unambiguous, clear and addresses only a single issue. The list of positive and negative research question is as follows:

- How do nurses care for dying patients?
- Are nurses good at interpersonal skills?
- What interpersonal skills do ward sisters identify as being important in dealing with distressed relatives?
- Does a nurse's academic ability affect her performance at the clinical level?
- How many patients on ward 'X' have sacral pressure sores of more than 2cm in diameter?
- Evaluate the impact of using Orem's Self Care model of nursing in the care of the elderly.
- What factors in nursing are perceived by ward staff as stressful?
- What is the ratio of trained to untrained nursing staff in this hospital?

What relevance do you think these problems have to your everyday work as a nurse? It is interesting to question the degree to which research questions and problems arise out of everyday nursing practice and the degree to which they are 'generated' by the person who sets out to undertake a research project. Should all nursing research address practical issues or should some research be carried out to clarify theoretical issues?

Evaluation: Check your results through with a tutor and discuss with him or her the problems of clarifying your own research question or problem. What are the constituents of a good research question? Were the research questions or problems clearly stated in the research projects you have read so far? Go back to one of them and try to extract such a question or problem.

As another level of evaluation, it is useful, before you finish the activity, to note down:

(a) what you learned from doing the activity,
(b) how you will use what you learned,
(c) how what you have learned relates to what you have read, and
(d) what you need to learn next.

Brainstorming

This a method of generating ideas, topics and issues that can later be clarified to form a cohesive plan. You will find the technique useful in at least the following situations:

- For clarifying a research question;
- For exploring potential research methods;
- For identifying possible constraints and solutions;
- For identifying new ideas for new projects;
- For problem-solving;
- For helping to identify material for an essay or project;
- For uncovering material for a teaching session;
- For sharing a wide range of ideas in a group setting;
- For developing creativity and intuition.

The Technique

1. On a sheet of paper write a heading that indicates the broad area that you wish to explore, e.g. 'Nursing' or 'Counselling' or 'Community Care'.
2. Under that heading and in no particular order, jot down everything that comes to mind when you think about that word. Do not omit anything and do not censor any words, phrases or sentences. Everything is to be jotted down. Continue this process until you have either filled the page or you can think of nothing else to write. The process may take anything from five minutes to one hour. The process may also be carried out in a group setting, when one person is elected to act as 'scribe' and who writes down the associations that other group members call out.
3. Now look through the list of words and phrases and strike out any that obviously are not immediately relevant. Be careful, though: you will be surprised how seemingly 'odd' ideas can lead you to a new perspective on the topic. This stage is a period of reflection on the 'free associations' that you have made in the previous stage. It is the stage in which

links start to be made between seemingly disparate ideas.

4. Finally, place your ideas and associations in an order of priority. In this way you bring structure to your thoughts. You may wish to develop a fairly elaborate system of headings and sub-headings or you may prefer only to cluster together certain related ideas. Either way, you will end the exercise with a wide range of ideas from which to work. Sometimes, you will end up with a huge number of ideas; at other times you will reach one single conclusion and that conclusion will very often be your real priority – even, if you are lucky, your research question itself.

5. Return to this list of ideas and phrases regularly and keep all the paper-work involved. In this way you can have a second period of reflection on the material and trace the development of your ideas as they evolve.

6. If the brainstorming procedure does help in the generation of a research question or problem, you will need to spend further time in refining the question or problem. This will usefully done in the company of another person who has had research experience.

Further Reading

Burnard, P. (1988) '"Brainstorming"': a practical learning activity in nurse education', *Nurse Education Today*, **8**, 354–8.

Burnard, P. and Morrison, P. (1993) *Survival Guide for Student Nurses*, Butterworth-Heinemann, Oxford.

de Bono, E. (1970) *Lateral Thinking: A Textbook of Creativity*, Penguin, Harmondsworth.

Ethical Considerations

'Ethics' is concerned with issues of 'right and wrong' and 'good and bad'. In research, ethical questions must be asked at all stages of the process. It is important to continue to ask questions such as:

- 'Is it right that I am asking people these questions in the process of doing my research?'
- 'Is what I am doing likely to harm anyone, physically, emotionally or socially?'
- 'Are my questions worth asking? Are they appropriate and/or important?'

We cannot assume that we have a right to undertake research or to ask questions of people, without gaining their permission or informed consent.

In order to protect people's rights in this area, most area health authorities have set up ethics committees which ask that researchers submit a copy of their research proposal to it for assessment regarding its ethical status. You must be clear about the ethical requirements and procedures in your district before you proceed beyond the planning stage with your research. Many district ethics committees will have a standard form that has to be filled in and submitted with the research proposal. The ethics committee may also ask to interview you about your proposal.

It is important not to overlook ethical issues when planning research. It is essential to discuss any proposals that you have (particularly if they involve asking for patient's cooperation) with a colleague, tutor or lecturer.

Further Reading

Burnard, P. and Chapman, C. (1993) *Professional and Ethical Issues in Nursing: The Code of Professional Conduct*, 2nd edn, Scutari, Chichester.
Medical Research Council (MRC) (1991) *The Ethical Conduct of Research on the Mentally Incapacitated*, MRC, London.
Royal College of Nursing (RCN) (1977) *Ethics Related to Research in Nursing*, RCN, London.

2.2   Writing a Research Proposal

By the end of this section you will have discovered:

• How to write a research proposal.

A research proposal is a detailed statement of what you intend to do, why you intend to do it and how you intend to go about it. It indicates both to you and anyone involved with your research both your ability to carry through the project and whether the design and methods you have selected are appropriate to the problem you have selected. The process of drawing up a research proposal can help you to further clarify your thoughts and methods. It is also necessary to give other people, outside of the project, the chance to examine your project and its methods. This is particularly true of those projects that required clearance through ethics committees. Any work involving patients will usually have to be considered by one or more such committees and those committees will always require you to submit a proposal. So, too, will any body that is considering giving you an award or offering you research money.

The process of drawing up a research proposal is often one that takes considerable time to get right. You may have to rough out various drafts and the people that you submit the proposal to may ask you to make various changes. Don't be put off by this but continue to work through the proposal making the required changes. Do not refuse to make changes recommended to you by those to whom you submit your work. If you do, you run the risk of supervision or support being withdrawn rather rapidly!

In the section 'Guidelines for a Research Proposal', below, you will find a structured outline for producing a research proposal. Note that this is only *one* way of drawing up such a proposal. Your school, college, awarding body or local authority may have another format. Even if it does, the basic structure of the proposal will always be similar to this.

Guidelines for a Research Proposal

1. Title of the project
2. Name and designation of the researcher
3. Supervisor
4. Department (school or college)
5. Statement of the problem
6. Aims and objectives of the project
7. Rationale for doing the research
8. Course of study being undertaken (if applicable)
9. Brief review of the pertinent literature
10. Research methods
11. Methods of analysis of data
12. Preparation of report
13. Ethical considerations
14. Costs involved (including itemised list and details of any funding bodies or details of self-funding)
15. Other considerations not covered in 1–12
16. Curriculum vitae of researcher (see Writing a Curriculum Vitae, below).

Further Reading

Calnan, J. (1984) *Coping with Research: The Complete Guide for Beginners*, Heinemann, London.
Darling, V.H. and Rogers, J. (1986) *Research for Practising Nurses*, Macmillan, London.
Hockey, L. (1985) *Nursing Research: Mistakes and Misconceptions*, Churchill Livingstone, Edinburgh.

Exercise 2.2

Aim of the exercise: To draw up a research proposal.

Planning stage: You can do this exercise on your own or in the company of a small group of colleagues, friends or students. Allow yourself plenty of time to complete the exercise and make notes of what you do, as you go. If you work with friends or colleagues, decide whether you will all carry out similar tasks or you will divide up the work between you.

Equipment / resources required: Notebook, pen and access to a nursing library.

What to do: Read through the research proposal outline, above, and make notes about your own research under those headings. Then continue to refine the proposal until you are content that it is clear, detailed and complete.

Evaluation: Show your proposal to a tutor and take note of any modifications that he or she may suggest. After you have written the proposal, ask yourself the following questions:

- Is the proposal realistic? Have I the necessary skills to undertake this piece of research? Have I the time to carry it through? Do I know how to undertake the various stages?
- Is the proposal clear? Have I used simple, unambiguous language and avoided unnecessary jargon?

Always explain technical terms, especially if the proposal is going to be read by lay people or those unfamiliar with research. Remember that your proposal may be provisional and require further amendments as you develop your thoughts and ideas. Bear in mind, too, that you may have to modify your proposal further as you progress through your projects. As we noted earlier, research can be a messy business and does not always go to plan. Sometimes, unexpected contingencies will force you to modify your plans.

- Have I covered each aspect of the proposal thoroughly?
- Does the proposal paint a complete word picture of what I intend to do and how I intend to do it?
- Can I anticipate any sections of the proposal which may cause others to be concerned or to ask questions.

Always be prepared for questions from other people, especially from supervisors and ethics committees.

As another level of evaluation, it is useful, before you finish the activity, to note down:

23

(a) what you learned from doing the activity,
(b) how you will use what you learned,
(c) how what you have learned relates to what you have read, and
(d) what you need to learn next.

Writing a Curriculum Vitae

There are many occasions, including when you are preparing a research proposal, when you will be required to present a curriculum vitae (CV). This should be typed, and should set out your 'life history' to date. Your CV gives the reader the opportunity to assess your suitability for undertaking the research you have planned. It also offers an insight into how you have studied and trained and the work what you have done to date. It is worthwhile investing time in the preparation of a CV and it is worthwhile keeping copies of it which can be updated from time to time. Headings that may be used to structure a CV include those below. It is usual to divide the CV up into sections for clarity of presentation and ease of reading. The headings are as follows:

CURRICULUM VITAE

Personal Details

Name

Home Address

Home Telephone Number

Nationality

Marital Status

Age

Date of Birth

Occupation

Work Address

Work Phone Number

Education

Schools and Colleges Attended (with dates)

Examinations Passed (with grades and dates)

Other Educational Achievements (awards, grants, scholarships, etc.)

Professional Training and Experience

Professional training (places, dates, qualifications obtained)

Posts Held (most recent first)

Present Post Held

Brief Outline of Responsibilities in Present Post

Salary and Point on the Scale

Professional Courses attended (management, refresher, etc.)

Publications and/or previous research

Hobbies and Interests

Other Details (e.g. driving license held, ability to type, other skills not discussed above).

If you work with a computer or word processor, it is worthwhile keeping a copy of your CV on disk and adding to it as your circumstances change.

2.3 Identifying Constraints

By the end of this section you will have discovered:

• What constraints are likely to affect your research.

Exercise 2.3

Aim of the exercise: To explore constraints as they apply to your project.

Planning stage: You can do this exercise on your own or in the company of a small group of colleagues, friends or students. Allow yourself plenty of time to complete the exercise and make notes of what you do, as you go. If you work with friends or colleagues, decide whether you will all carry out similar tasks or you will divide up the work between you.

Equipment / resources required: Notebook, pen and access to a nursing library.

What to do: Sit on your own and write down on a sheet of paper the headings contained in the table below. The structure of the table will allow you to identify any snags in your project and any things that may stand in the way of completing it. In the second column of the table, you are encouraged to use a problem-solving approach to identifying ways of dealing with the constraints that you have identified. You are then asked to plan action to help overcome any constraints. The process of doing the exercise will make the next stages of your project easier.

Table 2.1 Exploring possible constraints in your research project

Possible constraints	Suggestions for how constraints may be managed	Action
Brainstorm all possible constraints here. They may include such things as: • Other people's attitudes • Time factors • Financial limitations • Lack of specialist knowledge and skills about research.	Identify ideas for managing each constraint. Some constraints may be insurmountable but at least you will be prepared and you will be better able to plan to do next.	Write in here realistic things to be done and how you will do them.

Evaluation: What constraints did you identify? If you identified too many or too large constraints you may have to rethink part of your project and reduce your expectations. Discuss your findings with your colleagues and with a tutor and ask them to think about what they think may be constraints in your project. Be prepared to accept criticism and be prepared to adapt your strategy. This is another exercise that you can return to at various stages throughout the research process in order to plan ahead.

At this stage, you may want to consider the question of pilot testing your plan. A pilot study (as we will discuss later) is a small study to enable you to discover whether or not your proposed plan works well in practice. Discuss with your tutor whether or not this would be a good time to institute a pilot study. The pilot study can be an ideal way of uncovering practical and organisational problems. Once uncovered, these issues can be accounted for and your plan modified accordingly.

As another level of evaluation, it is useful, before you finish the activity, to note down:

(a) what you learned from doing the activity,
(b) how you will use what you learned,
(c) how what you have learned relates to what you have read, and
(d) what you need to learn next.

Conclusion

By now you should have prepared your initial proposal and be reasonably confident that you can carry it through. The more time that you spend in this process, the better, for it is preferable to iron out as many problems as you can early on rather than to have to make substantial changes later on.

Learning Check

If You are Working on Your Own

Read through the notes that you have kept whilst completing the exercises in this chapter and consider the following questions:

• What new knowledge have I gained?
• What new skills have I developed?
• How has my thinking about research changed?
• What do I need to do now?

Check that you have made reference cards for any new references that you have found whilst working on the exercises in this chapter.

If You are Working in a Small Group

Pair off and nominate one of you as A and one of you as B. For five minutes, A talks to B about what she has learned and B listens. This should *not* be a conversation: B's only role is to listen. After five minutes, roles are reversed and B talks to A about what she has learned and A listens. After the second five minutes, re-form into a group a discuss the experience.

If You are a Tutor and/or Facilitator

- Use the above pairs exercise with the group you are working with.
- Hold two 'rounds' in which each person in turn says *(a)* what she liked least about doing the activities and *(b)* what she liked most about doing the activities

3

Searching the Literature

Aims of this Chapter

- To explore literature resources;
- To discuss how to conduct a literature search;
- To consider how to review the literature critically;
- To encourage the writing of a literature review.

Introduction

This chapter focuses on the skills you will need in order to search for literature relevant to your project. A systematic search of the work already carried out in your field of interest is necessary so that you are clear about what has and what has not been done. You need to be conscientious and organised.

When you have completed the search, you will be able to:

- Summarise the previous research in your field of study and this will help you to formulate your own ideas/questions/problems;
- Have a better idea about what approaches and methods other researchers have used to study the area and you will be able to make an informed choice about the appropriateness of different procedures;
- Identify important omissions in the work that has already been completed and to design your study so that you are adding to the established body of knowledge. Also:
- You may wish to follow up published material by writing or phoning the author concerned to clarify issues raised in their work, to discuss possible lines of inquiry, or even to compliment them on the quality of their work!

Finally, it is worth noting that you must continue to search the literature throughout all the stages of the research process. Your field of study is constantly changing. You must keep up to date!

Bell, J. (1987) *Doing Your Research Project: A Guide for First-Time Researchers in Education and Social Science*, Open University Press, Milton Keynes, chs 3 and 4.

Cormack, D.F.S. (ed.) (1991) *The Research Process in Nursing*, 2nd edn, Blackwell, Oxford.

Haywood, P. and Wragg, E.C. (1982) *Evaluating the Literature: Rediguide 2: Guides in Educational Research*, Nottingham University, Nottingham.

Sharp, D. (1986) 'Searching health education literature: bibliographic and indexing tools', *Health Education Journal*, **45** (4) 239–42.

Stodulski, A.H. and Stafford, S.M. (1982) 'Disseminating research information in the UK: "Nursing Research Abstracts" from the "Index of Nursing Research"', *International Journal of Nursing Studies*, **19** (4) 231–6.

3.1 Exploring the Literature Resources

By the end of this section you will have discovered:

- Where to find information about previous work related to your field of study;
- The accessibility of using these sources from the points of view of time, energy and cost.

Exercise 3.1

Aim of the exercise: To identify literature resources.

Planning stage: You can do this exercise on your own or in the company of a small group of colleagues, friends or students. Allow your yourself plenty of time to complete the exercise and make notes of what you do, as you go. If you work with friends or colleagues, decide whether you will all carry out similar tasks or you will divide up the work between you.

Equipment / resources required: Notebook, pen and access to a nursing library.

What to do: Draw three concentric circles on a page (see the example in Figure 3.1). The inner circle represents literature resources that are immediately available (e.g. your own books,

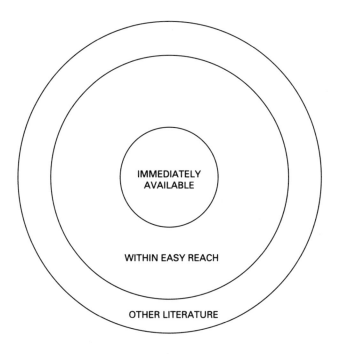

IMMEDIATELY
AVAILABLE

WITHIN EASY REACH

OTHER LITERATURE

Figure 3.1

journals, etc.). The middle circle represents those resources that are available within reasonably easy reach (e.g. school of nursing library, hospital library, public library, friends, colleagues, etc.). The outer circle represents those resources that are available through rather more application (e.g. inter-library loan scheme, microfiche copies, RCN literature search service, etc.). Personalise this diagram so that it becomes a source of reference for you when you do your literature searching. Add to it as you discover new sources of information. Keep it with you throughout your research project. You will often need it! Also, keep a list of the libraries and resource centres that you have visited and the sections in those departments that you have explored. In this way, you become more systematic in your search and avoid unnecessary repetition.

Evaluation: Go through the information contained in the three circles and identify which sources you are using at present. Write down on a sheet of paper those sources that you need more information about and write down those sources that you will use in the coming weeks. Do any of the sources charge for their services? If so, have you budgeted for this? Are any of the sources likely to take considerable time to respond to your request? If so, can you account for this in planning your work? If not, would it be better to seek this information from another source? Finally, do you really need this information: is it vital to your project? If you have doubts about this, talk to your supervisor about this piece of information. Much time can be lost searching out esoteric and obscure papers that only distantly relate to the project! Keep it simple: start with the obvious!

As another level of evaluation, it is useful, before you finish the activity, to note down:

(a) what you learned from doing the activity,
(b) how you will use what you learned,
(c) how what you have learned relates to what you have read, and
(d) what you need to learn next.

3.2 Finding and Summarising Relevant Literature

By the end of this section you will have discovered:

• How to find literature and information as part of your research project;
• How to keep records of the literature you find.

Guidelines for Evaluating Research Reports

As you go through the literature, you will find reports of other people's research. The following guidelines will help you to ask evaluative questions about that research. The guidelines will also help you to firm up your ideas about problems, methods and analytical techniques in your own research project.

1. The Research Problem
• Is the problem clearly stated?
• Is the problem researchable?
• Does the problem relate directly to nursing?

2. The Literature Review
• Is the review of the literature relevant to the topic?
• Is it comprehensive?
• How current are the sources of literature?
• Is the referencing method used correctly?

- Is the review laid out logically?
- Is a summary offered at the end of the review that spells out implications for the present study?

3. Design of the Study
- Is there a statement of the overall design of the study?
- Is there a discussion about the theoretical framework of the study?
- If hypotheses are offered, are they unambiguous and clearly stated?
- Is there a clear description of:
  (a) what the researcher planned to do?
  (b) what the researcher did?
  (c) how the researcher did it?
- Are relevant technical terms defined clearly?

4. Data Collection
- Is the data collection method described clearly?
- Does the researcher justify the use of her method?
- Is the sample discussed in terms of relevance and size?
- Are the instruments used for data collection clearly described?
- Are the issues of reliability and validity addressed? (These are discussed in Chapter 6 of this book.)
- Is there a clear description of what the researcher did when she collected the data?

5. Data Analysis
- Are the methods of analysis appropriate for the data?
- Are those methods clearly described?
- Is the presentation of findings clearly laid out (in tables, graphs, pie charts, etc.)?
- Is there adequate discussion of the results and findings?

6. Conclusions and Recommendations
- Are the conclusions that the researcher makes justified?
- Are the conclusions linked sufficiently with the researcher's original purpose?
- Are the recommendations practical?
- Has the researcher discussed the implications for further research?
- Has the researcher discussed the limitations of the study?

Further Reading

Morrison, P. (1991) 'Critiquing research', *Surgical Nurse*, **4** (3) 20–2.
Ogier, M. (1989) *Reading Research: Or How to Make Research More Approachable*, Scutari, London.
Phillips, L.R.F. (1986) *A Clinician's Guide to the Critique and Utilization*

of Nursing Research, Appleton-Century-Crofts, Norwalk, Connecticut.
Ward, M.J. and Fetler, M.E. (1979) 'What guidelines to be followed in critically
evaluating research reports?', *Nursing Research*, **28** (2) 120–6.

Reviewing Other Literature

Apart from reviewing research reports, you will want to read other sorts of
literature including: theoretical discussion in journals and books, biographi-
cal literature, discussion of methodology and technique, textbooks, policy
documents, official reports and sometimes fiction.

As you read, consider the following:

- Are arguments expressed clearly?
- Are they substantiated by either:
  (a) reference to research or
  (b) rational argument?
- Are the assumptions underlying an argument spelt out?
- Are the limitations of a particular argument identified?
- Does the author have a particular position to state which blinds him to
  other possibilities?
- Is the discussion balanced and informed or is it polemical?
- If rational argument is used, does it flow in a logical and ordered manner?
- Are the arguments relevant to your subject area?
- Does the author use technical terms and if so does he explain what he
  means by his use of them?
- Could you summarise the main points of argument?
- Have other authors that you have read expressed different views? Could
  you summarise them?
- Do you agree with what the author says? If so, why? If not, why?

This is not an exhaustive list of possible issues to be explored when reading
literature other than research reports but it will help you to evaluate what
you read and to become more critical of your reading.

Further Reading

Brink, P.J. and Wood, M.J. (1988) *Basic Steps in Planning Nursing Re-
search: From Question to Proposal*, Jones & Bartlett, Boston, MA.
LoBiondo-Wood, G. and Haber, J. (1990) *Nursing Research: Methods, Critical
Appraisal and Utilisation*, 2nd edn, Mosby, St Louis.

Exercise 3.2

Aim of the exercise: To find a specific piece of information from a library.

Planning stage: Prepare to go to a library which contains a reasonable selection of books and journals on nursing. Allow yourself plenty of time to complete the exercise and make notes of what you do, as you go.

Equipment/resources required: Notebook, pen and access to a nursing library, transport.

What to do: Go to the library and ask the librarian to explain the cataloguing system to you. Find the following publications or articles, using the cataloguing system and make notes of how and where you found them. Note the library cataloguing number on the spine of the book. This information will be important for the next exercise!

Field, P.A. and Morse, J.M. (1985) *Nursing Research: The Application of Qualitative Approaches*, Croom Helm, London.
Fielding, R.G. and Llewelyn, S.P. (1987) 'Communication training in nursing may damage your health and enthusiasm: some warnings', *Journal of Advanced Nursing*, **12**, 281–90.

Evaluation: What, if any, problems did you have in using the cataloguing system? What was the name of the cataloguing system (e.g. the Dewey system) used in that library? Did you ask the librarian to find the publications for you? If you did, will you know your way around the library next time? How did you record the information about where the publications were?

As another level of evaluation, it is useful, before you finish the activity, to note down:

(a) what you learned from doing the activity,
(b) how you will use what you learned,
(c) how what you have learned relates to what you have read, and
(d) what you need to learn next.

Abstracts

Remember not to be too narrow in your search for relevant literature. Consider consulting abstracting indexes in the social, biological and behavioural sciences, as well as those in nursing. Examples of interesting references in these fields include:

Applied Social Science Index and Abstracts (ASSIA)
Dissertation Abstracts International
Health Service Abstracts
Midwifery Research Database (MIRAID)
Nursing Abstracts
Nursing Research Abstracts
Psychological Abstracts
Quality Assurance Abstracts
Social Science Abstracts
Sociological Abstracts
Sociology of Education Abstracts

Computerised Abstracting Services

Consider, also, the growing number of computerised abstracting services. Your local library may be able to organise a computer search of the literature. However, they can be costly, they can generate many unwanted references and they are not a replacement for conventional forms of literature searching.

A variety of CD-ROMs (Compact Disk: Read Only Memory) are available which list research reports and abstracts in a similar way to the abstracts identified above. The big advantage of the CD-ROM system is the huge amount of information that is contained on each disk. Also, CD-ROMS can be very quickly searched and you only need to select out the references that you need. Ask your librarian for details about how to use this services. You may need some training to use the system, at first. Once you are familiar with the technology, you will be able to do searches easily and quickly. Also, if you have a computer at home, you can download your searches to floppy disk, take them home, and browse through your selection.

A variety of CD-ROMS are available and these are some of the ones most useful to health professionals. All of these and a wide range of other CDs and CD-ROM drives are available, in the UK, from Microinfo Ltd, CD-ROM Division, PO Box 3, Omega Park, Alton, Hampshire, GU34 2PG. The names in brackets refer to the publishers of these compact disks.

- *The British Medical Journal 1986–1990* (Macmillan). Selections from one of the most important medical journals.
- *The Lancet 1986–1990* (Macmillan). This includes the complete text of articles from the Lancet between these years.
- *Martindale: The Extra Pharmacopoeia*. This is the complete text on disk and it is updated quarterly.

- *Oxford Textbook of Medicine* (Oxford University Press). This is the electronic edition of a standard text.
- *Cumulative Index to Nursing and Allied Health Literature* (Cambridge Scientific Abstracts). The CINAHL provides access to virtually all English language nursing journals, publications from the American Nurses' Association, the National League for Nursing and primary journals in more that a dozen allied health disciplines.
- *Compact Library: AIDS* (Macmillan). This is a collection of clinical information on all aspects of AIDS treatment, research and patient management.
- *Medline* (Cambridge Scientific Abstracts) This provides access to worldwide biomedical literature and will be well known to many health care professionals.
- *Micromedix – Computerised Clinical Information System* (Micromedex Inc.) Micromedex Inc. is an established publisher of evaluated patient care information.
- *PsycLit* (Silver Platter). This series of compact disks contains citations to over 1,300 journals in psychology and the behavioural sciences.
- *Sociofile* (Silver Platter). This is an index to and abstracts of the literature of sociology from 1,800 journals published worldwide.

Further Reading

Burnard, P. (1993) *Personal Computing for Health Professionals*, Chapman & Hall, London.
Koch, W. and Rankin, J. (eds) (1987) *Computers and their Applications in Nursing*, Harper & Row, London.

3.3 Keeping a Card Reference System

By the end of this section you will have discovered:

- How to keep a record of what you read;
- How to organise these records.

Exercise 3.3

Aims of the exercise: To demonstrate how you can make useful notes from what you read, and how to organise these notes.

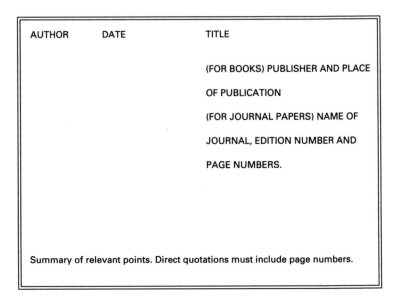

AUTHOR	DATE	TITLE
		(FOR BOOKS) PUBLISHER AND PLACE OF PUBLICATION (FOR JOURNAL PAPERS) NAME OF JOURNAL, EDITION NUMBER AND PAGE NUMBERS.

Summary of relevant points. Direct quotations must include page numbers.

Figure 3.2   Example layout of an index card

Planning stage: You will need access to your library again. Allow yourself plenty of time to complete the exercise and make notes of what you do, as you go.

Equipment required: Index cards (13 x 7.5 cms), a box for filing the cards in, a pen.

What to do: Go to your library and find the article by Fielding and Llewelyn (1987), and the book by Field and Morse (1985), detailed in the previous exercise, and then attempt to answer the following questions:

(a) What factors hamper the development of communications training in the Fielding and Llewelyn (1987) paper?
(b) What is the purpose of qualitative research according to Field and Morse (1985)?

Llewelyn, S.P. and Trent, R.7. 1987   Nursing in the Community,
                                        British Psychological Society,
                                        Methuen London

Useful chapter on sex and the patient (pp 83–97).
Discussion of caring for the elderly person in the community.
'. . . how people behave and feel in sickness and distress can only really be
understood if you also know about their current life situations and what
their background is'. (p. 4)

Figure 3.3   Example of a completed index card

Once you have answered the questions you will need to make an accurate record of what the authors have said in support of your answers. Details about the sources of your literature are required so that your project can be written up and referenced accurately. We recommend that you use the following system.

Prepare your index cards in the format illustrated in Figures 3.2 and 3.3. By all means tailor the layout to suit your own needs but once you have settled on a format, stick to it. Always carry some index cards around with you, so that when you find a new and relevant reference, you can make notes about it, there and then. Note that under copyright laws, you cannot make photocopies of book pages and articles, so make sure that your referencing system is thorough.

Evaluation: You may have been tempted to use the author's words to answer the questions, but it is more useful to make your own synopsis of the article or book. Use quotations sparingly and remember to keep quotations in inverted commas, and record the precise page number. Keep your cards in alphabetical order in a plastic box. Consider, also, cross-referencing cards and/or placing them together in sections under subject headings, e.g.: 'community nursing', 'nursing process', 'nursing models', etc.

As another level of evaluation, it is useful, before you finish the activity, to note down:

(a) what you learned from doing the activity,
(b) how you will use what you learned,
(c) how what you have learned relates to what you have read, and
(d) what you need to learn next.

Computerised Reference Databases

If you have a computer, you may want to keep your reference collection on it. You have two options here: you can either list all your references in a single, word processor file, or you can store them in a database program.

The simplest approach is the first one. You simply open a word processing file and then put your references into it, in the form of paragraphs, as you collect them. If your word processor has a 'sorting' facility, it doesn't matter what 'order' you type them in. Once you have put in new references, you get the program to sort the entire list into alphabetical order. Here is an example of what your file will look like.

Brown, P.J. (1991) *Essential Biology*, Arnold & Smith, London.
Smith, D. (1992) *Nursing for Professionals*, Chapman & Hall, London.
Watson, P. (1990) 'A study of the way in which pressure sore care has been conducted in three London teaching hospitals', *Journal of Nursing Studies*, **2** (34) 36–45.

There are many advantages to this approach to storing references. First, you can add new ones to the file very easily. Second, you can easily 'cut and paste' references from your list straight into your essay or project. Third, the whole system is very easy to use and administer. If you feel that you will not be collecting huge numbers of references, this system may suit you.

The second approach is to use a ready written database program. There are at least three sorts of these:

- A bibliographical database program.
- A flat file database program.
- A free-form database program.

The bibliographical database program is one that is specially written for recording references. Thus, the program is set up for you to enter names, dates, titles and publishers of books and the details of journal papers. Such programs are usually fairly easy to run and you can transfer references from your word processor into the program and export references into your essays

40

and projects. The problem with using such a program is that it may not be possible to set it up *exactly* as you would like it.

This is where a flat file database program may be useful. This sort of program is flexible and works on the principle of 'forms and fields'. A 'form' is the equivalent of a single card, on which you keep the details of your reference. A 'field' is a space on that form in which you store specific details (author, date, title, publisher).

Before you can use a database of this sort, you must first determine what fields you need and how *long* each of the fields will be. The best way to do this is to draw an example form, on paper, before you switch on the computer. You also need to make sure that each of your fields is long enough to contain the longest piece of text you are likely to put in it. Some flat file database systems insist that you can insert a maximum of 255 characters in any given field. This is usually long enough for most purposes but it does mean that you have to be careful about the length of the 'comments' that you write.

A flat file database system allows you to store you references systematically and allow you to design your own system to suit yourself. A number of commercial systems are available including *Paradox and Superbase*. All take a little time to 'learn' and to get used to but such time is well invested.

The free-form database program overcomes the limitations of the flat form variety. The free-form program does not use forms and fields. Instead, you simply type all of your text into the program and then, at a later date, you search for the text you have typed. Thus, you may search for the word 'counselling' and the program will call up all the books and journal papers that have 'counselling' in the title. Alternatively, you may search for 'Smith, P.J.' and the program will show you all the entries you have made under that name.

Again, there is a variety of free-form database programs available, such as *Memory Mate* and *Info Select*. One of the bonuses of both Memory Mate and Info Select is that they are also 'Terminate and Stay Resident' programs. That is to say that they can be made to 'pop up' over any other program you are using. Thus, you may be working in your word processor and you can call up Memory Mate to search for a particular reference. You can then 'cut and paste' that reference from Memory Mate directly into your word processing file. You can then 'close down' Memory Mate and return to work on your original document.

3.4   Critically Reviewing the Literature

By the end of this section you will have discovered:

• How to review what you read critically.

41

Exercise 3.4

Aim of the exercise: To explore styles of critical literature reviewing.

Planning stage: Negotiate access to a library that will be able to supply you with the articles referred to below. Allow time for reading and writing comments. Make notes as you go.

Equipment/resources required: Notebook, pen and access to a nursing library, transport.

What to do: Read the literature review sections of the following two articles. Compare the two styles of reviewing and note how each author uses references to other work. Note, too, whether or not they are critical of other people's work. It is important that reviews of the literature do not become lists of other people's research or theories!
Points to look for as you read:

- Does the author break the review up into sections?
- Does he/she question the methodology of previous research?
- Does he/she challenge the assumptions that previous writers make?
- Do you understand the points that are made?
- Is the review interesting?
- How recent is the literature referred to in the review?
- Is the review balanced: 'critical' doesn't just mean 'criticise'!
- Does the author have a particular axe to grind: philosophical, political, ideological?

Keep asking questions about what you are reading. Don't take what the writer says for granted. Challenge what is written and look for reasons for and explanations of the writer's arguments. To do this is to begin the process of critical evaluation. Note, however, that to be 'critical' is not only to pick holes in the work nor to see it only in a negative light. To be critical is also to be able to discriminate between the 'good' as well as the 'bad' parts of the work.
The two articles for consideration are:

Goodman, C. (1986) 'Research on the informal carer: a selected literature review', *Journal of Advanced Nursing*, **11** 705–12.
McCloskey, J.C. (1981) 'The effects of nursing education on job

effectiveness: an overview of the literature', *Research in Nursing and Health*, **4**, 355–73.

Complete an index card for each of these articles and make notes on those cards about the content of the two papers. In this way you will reinforce the habit of keeping notes of your reading.

Evaluation: Read through your notes, consider your summaries and then ask a colleague to read one of the papers and discuss your individual views. Note how different people's perceptions of the same paper can vary considerably!

As another level of evaluation, it is useful, before you finish the activity, to note down:

(a) what you learned from doing the activity
(b) how you will use what you learned,
(c) how what you have learned relates to what you have read, and
(d) what you need to learn next.

3.5 Writing a Literature Review

By the end of this section you will have discovered:

• How to write your own literature review.

Writing a Literature Review

The point about writing up a literature review is not simply to list all the books and papers that you have read about the particular topic in question but to do so *critically*. You also need to *organise* the review under a range of headings. It is important that a literature review should 'flow' and that it takes the reader through a series of sections that are logical and orderly. The overall aim of the literature review is to place your piece of research in context. It should answer the following questions:

• What research has been done prior to this study?
• Why is this field of study of interest?
• What are some of the problems associated with this field?
• How is the field organised?
• What are the main theories, arguments, research designs, modes of analysis used in the field?

- How does all this link with the *larger* field of nursing?
- What new issues, needing to be addressed, have emerged from your search of the literature?
- What are the recommended approaches for dealing with these issues?

A good literature review should take into account the following points.

- It should be comprehensive and up to date.
- It should be clearly structured with good use made of headings and sub-headings.
- It should be a *critical* account of previous work carried out in the field.
- It should be appropriately and accurately referenced.

Further Reading

Brearley, S. (1990) *Patient Participation: The Literature*, Scutari, London.
Choppin, R.G. (1983) *The Role of the Ward Sister: A Review of the British Literature since 1987*, King's Fund Centre, London.
Cooper, H.M. (1984) *The Integrative Research Review: A Systematic Approach*, Sage, London.

Exercise 3.5

Aim of the exercise: To undertake a short literature review.

Planning stage: Identify a topic of your choice. Identify the literature resources relevant to your chosen area. Arrange access to your local library.

Equipment required: Index cards, box for keeping the cards in, pen, transport.

What to do: Go to your library and find 10 articles or books related to your chosen subject area. Make a summary of each of these on the index cards, which should, of course, contain full details of the references. Then write a critical review of the ten articles of not more than 500–1000 words.

Evluation: Choose one of the following options:

(a) Show the review to your tutor or supervisor;
(b) Ask friends or colleagues to read and comment on it;
(c) Share the review with a group of colleagues who have also undertaken the exercise.

As another level of evaluation, it is useful, before you finish the activity, to note down:

(a) what you learned from doing the activity,
(b) how you will use what you learned.
(c) how what you have learned relates to what you have read, and
(d) what you need to learn next.

You have now carried out one stage of the research process!

Conclusion

You should now be able to collect information relating to your area of interest and record the details of that information on index cards. You should also be developing an awareness of how to read and write a 'critical' literature review. Continue to read around these subjects and then move on to the next chapter in which we explore different approaches to research methodology. The skills learnt in this stage of the research process will be called upon time and time again throughout the development of your project.

Learning Check

If You are Working on Your Own

Read through the notes that you have kept whilst completing the exercises in this chapter and consider the following questions:

- What new knowledge have I gained?
- What new skills have I developed?
- How has my thinking about research changed?
- What do I need to do now?

Check that you have made reference cards for any new references that you have found whilst working on the exercises in this chapter.

If You are Working in a Small Group

Pair off and nominate one of you as A and one of you as B. For five minutes, A talks to B about what she has learned and B listens. This should *not* be a conversation: B's only role is to listen. After five minutes, roles are reversed and B talks to A about what she has learned and A listens. After the second five minutes, re-form into a group a discuss the experience.

If You are a Tutor and/or Facilitator

- Use the above pairs exercise with the group you are working with.
- Hold two 'rounds' in which each person in turn says *(a)* what she liked least about doing the activities and *(b)* what she liked most about doing the activities.

4

Approaches to Research Methodology

Aims of this Chapter

These are:

- To list the distinguishing characteristics between quantitative and qualitative methods of research;
- To discriminate between descriptive and experimental research;
- To identify the problems associated with subjectivity and objectivity;
- To help you consider which approach or series of approaches may best help you in your enquiry.

Introduction

As we have noted, there are different approaches to thinking about and doing research. Sometimes it is useful to count and categorise things. At other times it is instructive to find out how people perceive things. This chapter explores some differences between various approaches to research. The temptation to polarise thinking into approaches being 'either/or', is a strong one. We hope that in looking at the different concepts involved in this chapter you will come to see the various approaches as complimentary rather than competitive.

What You Need to Read

This should include the following:

Bryman, A. (ed.) (1988) *Doing Research in Organisations*, Routledge, London.
Cannon, C. (1989) 'Social research in stressful settings: difficulties for the

sociologist studying the treatment of breast cancer', *Sociology of Health and Illness*, **11** (1) 62–77.

Cormack, B.F.S. (ed.) (1984) *The Research Process in Nursing*, Blackwell, Oxford.

Dixon, B.R., Bouma, G.D. and Atkinson, G.B.J. (1987) *A Handbook of Social Science Research: A Comprehensive and Practical Guide for Students*, Oxford University Press, Oxford.

Field, P.A. and Morse, J.M. (1985) *Nursing Research: The Application of Qualitative Approaches*, Croom Helm, London.

Gilbert, N. (ed.) (1993) *Researching Social Life*, Sage, London.

Morgan, G. and Smircich, L. (1980) 'The Case for Qualitative Research', *Academy of Management Review*, **5** (4) 491–500.

Reason, P. and Rowan, J. (1981) *Human Inquiry: A Sourcebook of New Paradigm Research*, Wiley, Chichester, ch 1 and 2.

Skevington, S. (ed.) (1984) *Understanding Nurses: The Social Psychology of Nursing*, Wiley, Chichester.

4.1 The Differences Between Quantitative and Qualitative Research

By the end of this section you will have discovered:

• What the two words mean;
• How various writers define the distinction between the two in research;
• Some examples of quantitative and qualitative research.

Exercise 4.1

Aim of the exercise: To define the words 'quantitative' and 'qualitative'.

Planning stage: This exercise can be carried out either by the individual working on her own or by a group of people working together. Allow yourself plenty of time to complete the exercise and make notes of what you do, as you go. If you work with friends or colleagues, decide whether you will all carry out similar tasks or you will divide up the work between you.

Equipment/resources required: Notebook, pen and access to a nursing library.

What to do: Find three of the references referred to above. Find out how those writers use the words quantitative and qualitative. Then look up those words in the *Concise Oxford Dictionary* and notice any difference in usage between the dictionary and the usage of words in the research literature. How useful are dictionary definitions when considering the ways words are used in research?

Evaluation: Discuss the various definitions of the two approaches and consider how you may draw out characteristics that distinguish the two approaches from one another.

As another level of evaluation, it is useful, before you finish the activity, to note down:

(a) what you learned from doing the activity,
(b) how you will use what you learned,
(c) how what you have learned relates to what you have read, and
(d) what you need to learn next.

Exercise 4.2

Aim of the exercise: To identify the characteristics that differentiate quantitative and qualitative approaches to research.

Planning stage: Prepare to go to a library which contains a reasonable selection of books on research and nursing research. This activity can be carried out alone or in a small group. Allow yourself plenty of time to complete the exercise and make notes of what you do, as you go. If you work with friends or colleagues, decide whether you will all carry out similar tasks or you will divide up the work between you.

Equipment/resources required: Notebook, pen and access to a nursing library.

What to do: Look through and read sections of books on research and nursing research and complete the grid outlined in Figure 4.1. The grid offers you certain criteria for distinguishing between the practical differences between the two approaches. It also asks you to find three examples of quantitative and three examples of qualitative research from the nursing research literature. If you are working in a group, in your plenary session, try to think of other ways in which the two methods differ.

Characteristics	Quantitative research	Qualitative research
Purpose of the study		
Sample size		
Data collection methods		
Data analysis methods		
Method of presenting findings		
Three examples from the nursing literature		

Figure 4.1   Grid for comparing approaches

Evaluation: Discuss these lists with a colleague or with the group that you are working with and compare what they have to say about the differences between the two approaches and you own work. Is it possible to make a clear distinction between the two? What types of research problems lend themselves to the different approaches? Have any nursing research studies used both approaches?

As another level of evaluation, it is useful, before you finish the activity, to note down:

(a) what you learned from doing the activity,
(b) how you will use what you learned,
(c) how what you have learned relates to what you have read, and
(d) what you need to learn next.

Quantitative Research

Although definitions of quantitative research vary, quantitative approaches usually incorporate some or all of the following features:

- Adopts an underlying philosophy of *positivism*. This is a word you should look up and be clear about.
- Attempts to establish *laws* and general principles.
- Counts things and uses statistics to make sense of the data that are gathered.
- Makes use of experiments and develops hypotheses.
- Uses laboratory tests.
- Uses psychometric scales and structured tests.
- Employs validity and reliability tests.

Recommended Reading

Bowling, A. (1991) *Measuring Health: A Review of Quality of Life Measurement Scales*, Oxford University Press, Oxford.

McLaughlin, F.E. and Marascuilo, L.A. (1990) *Advanced Nursing and Health Care Research: Quantification Approaches*, W.B. Saunders, Philadelphia.

Reid, N. and Boor, J. R.P. (1987) *Research Methods and Statistics in Health Care*, Edward Arnold, Sevenoaks.

Qualitative Research

Although definitions of qualitative research vary, qualitative approaches usually incorporate some or all of the following features:

- Adopts a phenomenological perspective. This is another term that you should look up and become familiar with.
- Attempts to investigate personal understanding and meaning systems.
- Uses small samples.
- Is concerned with *interpretation* rather than *quantification*.
- Often involves in depth interviews, observation and the exploration of personal documents.
- Is person-centred rather than subject-centred.
- Uses different tests for reliability and validity than is the case with quantitative methods.

Recommended Reading

Giorgi, A. (1970) *Psychology as a Human Science: A Phenomenologically Based Approach*, Harper & Row, New York.

Morse, J.M. (ed.) (1989) *Qualitative Nursing Research: A Contemporary Dialogue*, Sage, London.

4.2 Descriptive and Experimental Research

By the end of this section you will have discovered:

• The differences between descriptive and experimental research

Exercise 4.3

Aim of the exercise: To identify the differences between descriptive and experimental research.

Planning stage: This exercise can be carried out either by the individual working on her own or by a group of people working together. Allow yourself plenty of time to complete the exercise and make notes of what you do, as you go. If you work with friends or colleagues, decide whether you will all carry out similar tasks or you will divide up the work between you.

Equipment/resources required: Notebook, pen and access to a nursing library.

What to do: Read the following four research reports which illustrate some different approaches to doing research:

Bogdan, R., Brown, M.A. and Foster, S.B. (1982) 'Be honest but not cruel: staff/patient communication on a neonatal unit', *Human Organisation*, **41** (1) 6–16.
Burnard, P. and Morrison, P. (1988) 'Nurses' perceptions of their interpersonal skills: a descriptive study using six category intervention analysis', *Nurse Education Today*, 8, 266–72.
Haywood, J. (1975) *Information, A Prescription Against Pain*, RCN, London.
Luker, K.A. (1982) *Evaluating Health Visiting Practice*, RCN, London.

Now answer the following questions:

• What methods did each of the studies use?
• What sort of information was collected in each of the studies?

- How was the data analysed?
- What, if any, generalisations were made by the researchers?

Now read the next section, 'Descriptive and Experimental Research', which identifies some differences in approach between descriptive and experimental research. Which type of approach was used in the four studies?

Evaluation: Check your decisions about the above studies with a colleague or a tutor.
   As another level of evaluation, it is useful, before you finish the activity, to note down:

(a) what you learned from doing the activity,
(b) how you will use what you learned,
(c) how what you have learned relates to what you have read, and
(d) what you need to learn next.

Descriptive and Experimental Research

There are many differences between descriptive and experimental research and they often depend on differences of belief about the nature of the person. For example, a person drawn to experimental research may believe that there are numerous similarities between people or that people's behaviour is causally determined. On the other hand, a person drawn to descriptive research may be more interested in just describing a place, situation or environment, believing that what is important in research is to note people's varying perceptions of the world. What we believe about the world will affect how we study it. Our beliefs about the nature of the world and of the people that inhabit it will affect:

- The sorts of questions we ask;
- The way we approach planning our research;
- The sorts of research methods we use;
- The way we interpret the data we collect;
- The conclusions we draw from our findings.

Further Reading

Dumas, R. (1987) 'Clinical trials in nursing', *Recent Advances in Nursing*, **17**, 108–25.
Hicks, C.M. (1990) *Research and Statistics: A Practical Introduction for Nurses*, Prentice-Hall, New York.

Wilson-Barnett, J. (1991) 'The experiment: is it worthwhile?', *International Journal of Nursing Studies*, **28** (1) 77–87.

Points of Debate in Research

For a number of years, there has been a debate about the pros and cons of quantitative and qualitative approaches to research. Some have seen this as a debate about *method* – about how to *do* research. Others have argued that it is a debate about what assumptions we make about human beings. The debate, however, is broader than just the quantitative/qualitative divide (and sometimes this is *not* a divide at all: some writers and researchers have argued that it is possible to *combine* the approaches). Hammersley offers a useful list of some of the points that are often raised when people argue about different approaches to research. The list may be useful in debates that *you* have about the topic:

1. Qualitative versus quantitative data;
2. The investigation of natural versus artificial settings;
3. A focus on meanings rather than on behaviour;
4. Adoption or rejection of natural science as a model;
5. An inductive versus a deductive approach;
6. Identifying cultural patterns as against seeking scientific laws;
7. Idealism versus realism (Hammersley, 1992).

4.3 Subjectivity and Objectivity in Research

By the end of this section you will have discovered:

- Some of the differences between subjectivity and objectivity;
- Some of the problems associated with these two concepts.

Exercise 4.4

Aim of the exercise: To explore the problems of subjectivity and objectivity

Planning stage: The exercise needs to be carried out with a small group of friends or colleagues. Allow yourself plenty of time to complete the exercise and make notes of what you do, as you go. Decide whether you will all carry out similar tasks or you will divide up the work between you.

Equipment/resources required: Notebook, pen and access to a nursing library.

What to do:

1. Look up the words 'subjectivity' and 'objectivity' in a good dictionary (what do you class as 'good' in this context?) Then look at some books on research and read about how researchers have battled with the notions of subjectivity and objectivity.
2. With your colleagues, sit and write individual descriptions of the room you are in at present. Aim at writing about one page.
3. Read out your reports and decide:
   • whose description was most accurate?
   • whose was most objective?
   • whose was most interesting?
   • whose was most different to all the others?

Now hold a discussion on the topic of subjectivity and objectivity and try to answer the following questions:

• How can you attempt to be objective in research?
• Do you need to be?
• If so, why?
• Is objectivity possible?
• Is there a place in research for the subjective report?
• If so, what is that place?

Evaluation: Read through a research report and note the degree to which the researcher has addressed the issue of objectivity. A useful paper, here, is:

LeCompte, M.D. and Goetz, J.P. (1982) 'Problems of reliability and validity in ethnographic research', *Review of Educational Research*, **52** (1) 31–60.

As another level of evaluation, it is useful, before you finish the activity, to note down:

(a) what you learned from doing the activity,
(b) how you will use what you learned,
(c) how what you have learned relates to what you have read, and
(d) what you need to learn next.

4.5 Selecting or Blending the Approaches

As you have worked through this chapter you will have begun to address some of the complexities and ambiguities of the process of doing research. In order to make decisions about which approach to research you use, you will have to become fairly clear about your own beliefs about human beings and about how you view the world. Your personal philosophy will always affect the way you think and act. You cannot detach yourself from your area of study to the degree that you look on as an objective and detached observer. For a further discussion of this issue, read:

Bryman, A. (1988) *Quantity and Quality in Social Research*, Unwin Hyman, London.

Polit, D.F. and Hungler, B.P. (1989) *Essentials of Nursing Research: Methods, Appraisal and Utilization*, 2nd edn, Lippincott, Philadelphia.

Roberts, C.A. and Burke, S.O. (1989) *Nursing Research: A Quantitative and Qualitative Approach*, Jones & Bartlett, Boston.

The following exercise helps you to think about these two issues.
By the end of this section you will have discovered:

- More about yourself!
- More about how your own beliefs about people and the world influence the way that you do research.

Exercise 4.5

Aim of the exercise: To explore individual beliefs about the person and about research.

Planning stage: The activity can be carried out alone or with a group of other people. Allow yourself plenty of time to complete the exercise and make notes of what you do, as you go. If you work with friends or colleagues, decide whether you will all carry out similar tasks or you will divide up the work between you.

Equipment/resources required: Notebook, pen and access to a nursing library.

What to do:
(a) Take a few sheets of paper and write out, in note form, your beliefs about how people are. For instance, you may or may not believe some of the following and may wish to make

notes about how you agree or disagree with the statements. Write the piece fairly quickly, do not worry about 'style' and do not feel that the piece has to be an academic paper.

Some of the statements you may wish to agree or disagree with are:

- People are a product of their childhoods.
- A person's personality is shaped by society.
- A person is born with a certain personality.
- People are totally responsible for the way they are.
- God is responsible for the way people are.
- People can change themselves in fundamental ways.
- Most people are similar to most other people.
- We can measure people's behaviour.
- What a person does tells us what sort of person he is.
- People are basically aggressive by nature.
- People are born 'good': society corrupts them.
- People are born 'bad': they have to learn to be good.
- Events are causally linked.
- There is no absolute way of determining causality.
- All theories about people are open to question.
- People are subject to certain laws of human nature.

(b) If you are working in a group, discuss your writing and your beliefs about the nature of the person with your colleagues. If not, go through the paper and turn each of your statements into a question. Thus, if you have written: People are free to choose their lives, raise the question 'Are people free to choose their lives?' In this way, you begin to think critically about your own core beliefs and assumptions about people. Try, if you can, to argue against each of the questions and thus identify arguments that oppose your views.

(c) Now write out a short report of what you think are the functions and uses of research. Some of the things you may want to consider include the following:

- To add to the body of knowledge;
- To develop a greater understanding of people and the world;
- To attempt to predict the future;
- To enhance the environment;
- To contribute to other people's wellbeing;
- To create more interest in research, in the researcher;
- To disprove some theory;
- To test a theory;

- To understand another person's point of view;
- To inform practice;
- To satisfy course requirements;
- To challenge other people's theories or views of the world.

If you are working in a group, discuss these reasons and functions with the your colleagues. To what degree are your reasons for doing research coloured by your views about the nature of people?

Evaluation: Talk these things through with someone who has completed a research project. Ask them how their beliefs and values have changed during and after the process of undertaking research. Compare your views about people with your researcher colleague's views.

As another level of evaluation, it is useful, before you finish the activity, to note down:

(a) what you learned from doing the activity,
(b) how you will use what you learned,
(c) how what you have learned relates to what you have read, and
(d) what you need to learn next.

Conclusion

Until you addressed some of these basic questions about people and about research you have not clarified your motivation nor developed the ability to be critical about what you believe and think. Research has the interesting effect of challenging all our cherished beliefs and values. It may be a good idea to get some practice.

Learning Check

If You are Working on Your Own

Read through the notes that you have kept whilst completing the exercises in this chapter and consider the following questions:

- What new knowledge have I gained?
- What new skills have I developed?
- How has my thinking about research changed?
- What do I need to do now?

Check that you have made reference cards for any new references that you have found whilst working on the exercises in this chapter.

If You are Working in a Small Group

Pair off and nominate one of you as A and one of you as B. For five minutes, A talks to B about what she has learned and B listens. This should *not* be a conversation: B's only role is to listen. After five minutes, roles are reversed and B talks to A about what she has learned and A listens. After the second five minutes, re-form into a group a discuss the experience.

If You are a Tutor and/or Facilitator

- Use the above pairs exercise with the group you are working with.
- Hold two 'rounds' in which each person in turn says *(a)* what she liked least about doing the activities and *(b)* what she liked most about doing the activities

5

Choosing a Research Method

Aims of this Chapter

These are:

- To identify issues that help you to make decisions about methods;
- To identify how to find out about the range of methods available in order to make an informed decision;
- To clarify which method of data collection you aim to use in your project;
- To clarify how your data is going to be analysed after collection.

Introduction

By now you will have clarified your research question and will be considering ways of collecting data that will help you to answer that question. The next issue is that of deciding which is the most effective means of collecting that data. Before you go ahead and collect research data, you need to be clear about the method you are going to use to collect it. In a previous chapter we noted that there are a number of theoretical or philosophical considerations to be made about what sort of research you are doing, including the debate about quantitative versus qualitative research, the question of subjectivity and objectivity and so on. These issues will reappear when you come to selecting a method of data collection. By the end of this section you will be clearer about what sort of method you want to choose. Much will depend, of course, on what you want to find out!

One word of caution. It is vital that you are clear about how you will *process* your data when you have collected it. Most researchers will be able to tell you horror stories of people who have collected masses of data only to be able to sit back and wonder what to do with it! In planning your method of data collection, you must select your method of analysis.

What You Need to Read

Dixon, B.R., Bouma, G.D. and Atkinson, G.B.J. (1987) *A Handbook of Social Science Research: A Comprehensive and Practical Guide for Students*, Oxford University Press, Oxford, ch. 6.

Long, A.F. (1984) *Research into Health and Illness: Issues in Design, Analysis and Practice*, Gower, Aldershot.

Omery, A. (1983) 'Phenomenology: a method for nursing research', *Advances in Nursing Science*, **5** (2) 49–63.

Reason, P. and Rowan, J. (1981) *Human Inquiry: A Sourcebook of New Paradigm Research*, Wiley, Chichester, Introduction.

The Concept of Research Design

The term 'research design' is sometimes used to designate a particular approach to doing research. Three designs are commonly used:

- Survey
- Experiment
- Case Study.

The survey is a systematic gathering of information from a reasonably large sample of people, events, literature, records and so forth. The purpose of a survey is usually to identify general trends or patterns in data. Examples of surveys may include:

- Nurse's attitudes to smoking;
- The number of nurses trained as enrolled nurses, at a particular hospital, during a particular period;
- The incidence of particular illnesses in different parts of the country.

The experiment sets out to test out a hypothesis or a theory. Experimental research tries to establish causal links between a number of factors. Examples of experimental design may include:

- The effect of information-giving to patients on their rate of recovery from illness;
- The effectiveness of one drug rather than another in treating a particular disorder.

Experimental research tries to prove or disprove a relationship between two or more factors. Thus, in the first example above the researcher attempts to see whether or not giving information to patients about their illness and treatment makes a difference to those patients recovery rate from their illness. He does *not* set out to describe the *effects* of giving information – he is trying to establish a causal relationship between *(a)* the information and *(b)* the patient's rate of recovery. The experimental researcher uses two groups of subjects in his research: the experimental group (who, in the above experiment, receive information) and the control group (who would receive no information). In both groups, the samples are selected to ensure that they are similar in all important characteristics save the one being investigated. Thus a researcher carrying out the above study would select people for both groups in terms of similarity of age, socio-economic background, weight, medical history, amount of time spent with nursing staff and so forth. The single difference between the two groups would be that one group would be given the information (the experimental group) whilst the other group (the control) would not. In this way, the researcher would argue that he is ensuring that the one remaining difference (the information) did or did not affect the rate of recovery of the patients in these two groups.

The case study is a very detailed account of a small number of examples of a particular experience, event or situation. It may also be used to describe a small number of people and their experiences. The aim of the case study approach is to 'paint a picture', to supply a description of people's thoughts, feelings and perceptions. It does not set out to prove causal relationships nor test hypotheses in the way that experimental research does.

Examples, here, may be:

- A description of how patients with multiple sclerosis cope with their disability,
- An account of what it is like to train as a nurse during a three-year course,

There are other examples of research design that are not so frequently used in nursing. Examples of these are:

- Historical research;
- Philosophical research.

These examples of research design offer broad headings of particular approaches to research. Under each of these headings (and frequently overlapping between them) are a series of research methods: methods of collecting research data. It is those methods that are the subject of this and the following chapters.

Further Reading

de Vaus, D.A. (1991) *Surveys in Social Research*, 3rd edn, Unwin Hyman, London.

Polit, D.F. and Hungler, B.P. (1989) *Essentials of Nursing Research: Methods, Appraisal and Utilization*, 2nd edn, Lippincott, Philadelphia.

Schatzman, L. and Strauss, A.L. (1973) *Field Research: Strategies for a Natural Sociology*, Prentice-Hall, Englewood Cliffs, New Jersey.

5.1 Making Decisions About Methods

By the end of this section you will have discovered:

- Exactly what you want to find out
- What other people have found out in this field and what methods they have used to collect data.

Exercise 5.1

Aim of the exercise: To help you to state clearly what it is you want to find out in your research as a pre-requisite of selecting the most appropriate method.

Planning stage: You can do this exercise on your own or in the company of a small group of colleagues, friends or students. Allow yourself plenty of time to complete the exercise and make notes of what you do, as you go. If you work with friends or colleagues, decide whether you will all carry out similar tasks or you will divide up the work between you.

Equipment/resources required: Notebook, pen and access to a nursing library.

What to do:
1. Through a the processes of brainstorming, prioritisation and clarification, write *in one sentence* what your research is going to be about.
2. Having clarified your ideas, go to the library and find three studies that have already explored aspects of the field of study that interests you. From those studies answer these questions:
3. How did the researchers state the problem that they were researching?
4. In what ways were the problems stated in those projects similar to and different to your own?
5. What methods of data collection did they use?

6. In what ways will your research clarify the field or add to the body of knowledge?
7. Why are you choosing *this* problem?

Evaluation: Discuss your research statement and the answers to the above questions with colleagues and with a tutor. Has the exercise made you modify your original research statement in any way or has it confirmed your need to pursue that line of research?

As another level of evaluation, it is useful, before you finish the activity, to note down:

(a) what you learned from doing the activity,
(b) how you will use what you learned,
(c) how what you have learned relates to what you have read, and
(d) what you need to learn next.

5.2 Identifying the Range of Available Methods

By the end of this section you will have discovered:

• The range of research methods available to you

Exercise 5.2

Aim of the exercise: To allow you to consider the range of possible data collection methods that will help you to answer your research question.

Planning stage: You can do this exercise on your own or in the company of a small group of colleagues, friends or students. Allow yourself plenty of time to complete the exercise and make notes of what you do, as you go. If you work with friends or colleagues, decide whether you will all carry out similar tasks or you will divide up the work between you.

Equipment/resources required: Notebook, pen and access to a nursing library.

What to do: Look through the list of research methods in Figure 5.1. Beside each one, use the following code and mark the second column accordingly:

RESEARCH METHOD	
Questionnaire	
Interview	
Observation	
Critical incident technique	
Multiple sorting technique	
Delphi technique	
Q sort	
Use of existing scales (attitude scales, personality inventories, assessment scales etc.)	
Physiological measures	
Projective techniques	
Experiential research methods	
Action research	
Repertory grid technique	
Use of existing records	

Figure 5.1

1. Suited to my project;
2. Possibly suited to my project;
3. Unsuited to my project;
4. I do not have enough information about this method to make a decision.

For example, if you feel that the interview method is a suitable one for your project, you put a 1. in the second column. If you feel that the questionnaire method is unsuited to your project, you put a 4 in the second column. If you feel that you do not know enough about the Q sort technique, put a 5 in column 2 and so on.

Evaluation: On what basis did you make your decisions? Do you have enough information to choose your method, at this stage, or do you need to do further studying? What does this exercise tell you about some of the problems of collecting data? (The marks you awarded in the above column are data!) What could you do to analyse this data?

As another level of evaluation, it is useful, before you finish the activity, to note down:

(a) what you learned from doing the activity,
(b) how you will use what you learned,
(c) how what you have learned relates to what you have read, and
(d) what you need to learn next.

If you found that you did not have sufficient information about certain of the above methods to be able to make a decision, refer the bibliography at the end of this book for other texts and journal articles that will help you to understand these methods and assess their suitability.

5.3 Choosing your Data Collection Method

By the end of this section you will have discovered:

• How to choose a data collection method for your project.

Exercise 5.3

Aim of the exercise: To enable you to make a choice about the method you will use to collect your research data.

Planning stage: You can do this exercise on your own or in the company of a small group of colleagues, friends or students. Allow yourself plenty of time to complete the exercise and make notes of what you do, as you go. If you work with friends or colleagues, decide whether you will all carry out similar tasks or you will divide up the work between you.

Equipment/resources required: Notebook, pen and access to a nursing library.

What to do: Note the methods that you have selected out from the last exercise as being suitable for your project. Now ask yourself the following questions about each method in order to be more clear about the choice you are going to make:

1. Do I know enough about the method?
   (a) If Y, proceed to next item.
   (b) If N, go to the library, read more about the method, and discuss it with your tutor of someone who has had experience in this field OR proceed to next chapter.

2. Can I justify using this method rather than another?
   (a) If Y, proceed to next item.
   (b) If N, is this through lack of knowledge about other methods? If Y, read up on other methods. If N, proceed to next question in this chain. Is it because I could use a variety of methods? If Y, proceed to next item and keep a range of options open.

3. Have I got the skills to carry out the method?
   (a) If Y, proceed to next item.
   (b) If N, find out what the skills are from the library or from a tutor.

4. Is special equipment required to use this method?
   (a) If Y, have you access to it? If N, can you get access? If N, abandon this method.
   (b) If N, proceed to next item.

5. Does the method take considerable time to use?
   (a) If Y, have I got the time within my time schedule? If Y, proceed to next item. If N, abandon method.
   (b) If N, proceed to next item.

6. Does the method require a large sample? [Before answering this question, read around the question of sampling and discuss it with your tutor. Sampling is also explored in Chapter 6 of this book.]
   (a) If Y, Have I got access to the number required? If Y, proceed to next item. If N, abandon method.
   (b) If N, proceed to next item.

7. Do I know someone who has used this method and can give me support?

   (a) If Y, proceed to next item.

   (b) If N, Can I find someone? If Y, proceed with your project. If N, proceed with caution!

Evaluation: These are some of the questions that must be asked before you proceed with your project. Go to a tutor and ask them to quiz you on your chosen method. Ask a colleague to act as 'devil's advocate' and ask you particularly awkward questions about the method.

The final and most important question must be: Is this method the most appropriate one for answering your research question?

As another level of evaluation, it is useful, before you finish the activity, to note down:

(a) what you learned from doing the activity,

(b) how you will use what you learned,

(c) how what you have learned relates to what you have read, and

(d) what you need to learn next.

5.4   Choosing your Method of Data Analysis

By the end of this section you will have discovered:

• The appropriate method for your research project.

As we noted earlier, it is vital that you consider how you will analyse your data as your collect it. This decision must be made alongside the decision about which data collection method you are going to use and not after that decision.

Exercise 5.4

Aim of the exercise: To help you to select the most appropriate method of analysis for your data.

Planning stage: You can do this exercise on your own or in the company of a small group of colleagues, friends or students. Allow yourself plenty of time to complete the exercise and make notes of what you do, as you go. If you work with friends or colleagues, decide whether you will all carry out similar tasks or you will divide up the work between you.

Equipment/resources required: Notebook, pen and access to a nursing library.

What to do:
Consider the following questions: At the end of your project.

- Are you going to have data which is easily converted into numbers (e.g. A person may be asked to state whether they agree or disagree with a set of attitude statements in which the range of responses is: strongly disagree, disagree, uncertain, agree and strongly agree. These response labels can be given numerical values as follows: SD=1, D=2, UC=3, A=4, and SA=5. These numbers can then be totalled and statistic procedures used to identify trends in the data.)

OR

- Are you going to have data in the form of text or other 'blocks' of words (e.g. a series of interview transcripts or a series of passages taken from books, documents, records, etc.)?

OR

- Is your project likely to lead to the production of both numbers and text? If so, read and work through both of the sections below.

If your project will lead you to numbers, consider the following questions:

- Are you clear about how you will collect and store your data?
- Do you have the necessary skills to perform the mathematics required in processing the data?
- If statistical tests are required, do you know which ones they are and can you use them?
- Where can you obtain further statistical advice?
- Do you know how to interpret statistical data?
- Do you know the limitations of using figures as data?
- How will you present your figures when you write up your report?

Now read: Part Two, Selecting methods of data collection, in Bell, J. (1987) *Doing Your Research Project: A Guide for First-Time Researchers in Education and Social Science,* Open University, Milton Keynes.

If your project will lead you to the production of text, consider the following questions:

- Are you clear about how you will collect and store your data?
- Do you have the necessary skills to analyse and categorise the data?
- Where can you obtain further advice on handling textual data?
- What psychological, sociological or political theories will guide your analysis?
- Do you know how to interpret any findings?
- Do you know the limitations of using raw text as data?
- How will you present your data when your write up your report?

Now read: Turner, B.A. (1981) 'Some practical aspects of qualitative data analysis: one way of organising the cognitive processes associated with the generation of grounded theory', *Quality and Quantity,* 15, 225–47.

Evaluation: Discuss your work with your colleagues and with your tutor.
   As another level of evaluation, it is useful, before you finish the activity, to note down:

(a) what you learned from doing the activity,
(b) how you will use what you learned,
(c) how what you have learned relates to what you have read, and
(d) what you need to learn next.

Pilot Studies

Now that you have considered a variety of methods of collecting data, you will want to 'try out' one or more methods. This will usually lead you to doing a pilot study.
   A pilot study is a very small-scale version of the research project which allows you to test out your data collection method and allows you to preview the sort of data that the method will collect for you. It should point up deficiencies in your planning and development of the data collection method

and will enable you to smooth out such deficiencies. Alternatively, it may show you that the method you have chosen is not suitable for your project. In this case you may have to go back to the drawing board and consider other methods. Then, of course, you will have to conduct another pilot study. The details of the pilot study should always be written into your final research report.

Time spent at this stage can pay great dividends later on. Some of the questions that a pilot study will allow you to consider are:

- Can the respondents understand what is being asked of them?
- Does the data collection method collect the sort of data I want?
- Have I got time to use this method?
- Are there ethical problems associated with this method?
- Do I know how to analyse the data that this method generates?
- What revisions are required to modify my plan?

Further Reading

Lopez, M.J. and Radford, M.H. (1985) 'District nurse training: a pilot survey of demand, provision and students', *Journal of Advanced Nursing*, **10** (4) 361–7.

Prescott, P.A. and Soeken, K.L. (1989) 'The potential uses of pilot work', *Nursing Research*, **38** (1) 60–2.

Conclusion

You should now be more clear about how you want to conduct your research project. In the following chapters we will consider more closely the issues of method and analysis.

Learning Check

If You are Working on Your Own

Read through the notes that you have kept whilst completing the exercises in this chapter and consider the following questions:

- What new knowledge have I gained?
- What new skills have I developed?
- How has my thinking about research changed?
- What do I need to do now?

Check that you have made reference cards for any new references that you have found whilst working on the exercises in this chapter.

If You are Working in a Small Group

Pair off and nominate one of you as A and one of you as B. For five minutes, A talks to B about what she has learned and B listens. This should *not* be a conversation: B's only role is to listen. After five minutes, roles are reversed and B talks to A about what she has learned and A listens. After the second five minutes, re-form into a group a discuss the experience.

If You are a Tutor and/or Facilitator

- Use the above pairs exercise with the group you are working with.
- Hold two 'rounds' in which each person in turn says *(a)* what she liked least about doing the activities and *(b)* what she liked most about doing the activities

6

Methods of Collecting Data

Aims of this Chapter

- To explore common methods of data collection;
- To identify the strengths and limitations of each method;
- To enable you to consider the usefulness or otherwise of each of these methods for your own research project.

Introduction

In the last chapter we suggested ways that you might make decisions about how to collect data for your project. In this chapter we look at specific data collection methods. You will already have decided what methods you are likely to use but it may be useful to read through this chapter and do the exercises. This way you will familiarise yourself with other methods and you may find that you want to change your data collection method, either slightly or radically. If not, you will confirm that your original decision was right.

This chapter deals with those methods that are very well established in the research field. Traditional ways of finding out things have tended to be:

- Talking to people;
- Asking people to answer questions;
- Doing experiments;
- Going and seeing what's there.

Therefore, this chapter considers the following methods of data collection:

- Structured interviews
- Questionnaires

- Experiments
- Observation.

In the next chapter we will consider some other ways of collecting data.

Validity and Reliability

Two concepts central to the collection of data is that the methods used must be both **valid** and **reliable**. Stated simply, validity refers to whether or not a method measures what it sets out to measure, e.g. does an intelligence test really measure intelligence? Reliability refers to the issue of whether or not a method of measurement works consistently in producing similar results in similar situations, e.g. if an evaluation tool is used with this group of students at the end of this term, will it give me similar and comparable results when I use it with that group of students at the end of that term?

Summarising the two concepts, Gilbert offers the following illustration:

> researchers want their indicators to be as good as possible. This means that the measurements which they make should be **valid** (accurately measuring the concept) and **reliable** (consistent from one measurement to the next). For instance, suppose that you want to measure people's consumption of alcohol (a concept). You choose to do this using a questionnaire in which you will ask respondents to tell you how much they drank during the previous month. In fact, this is not a good indicator of alcohol consumption. People tend to under-report consumption – they say that they drink less than they actually drink – casting doubts on the validity of the indicator. Also, people have difficulty remembering in detail what they were doing as long as a month ago. This means that if you were to ask someone repeatedly over the course of a few days what they had drunk during the previous month it is quite likely that they would give you different answers, just because they were not remembering consistently. The indicator is not reliable (Gilbert, 1993).

There are different questions about validity and reliability to be addressed in using quantitative and qualitative approaches to research. Therefore, the reader is recommended to read the following references on the issues of validity and reliability. The issues of validity and reliability are so central to research that they will also crop up in nearly all books that you read about research.

Cook, T.D. and Campbell, D.T. (1979) *Quasi-Experimentation: Design and Analysis Issues for Field Settings*, Rand McNally, Chicago.
Le Compte, M.D. and Goetz, J.P. (1982) 'Problems of reliability and valid-

ity in ethnographic research', *Review of Educational Research*, **52** (1) 31–60.

Sapsford, R.J. and Evans, J. (1984) 'Evaluating a research report' in J. Bell, T. Bush, A. Fox, J. Goodey and S. Golding (eds) *Conducting Small-Scale Investigations in Educational Management*, Harper & Row, London.
Waltz, C.F., Strickland, O.L. and Lenz, E.R. (1984) *Measurement in Nursing Research*, F.A. Davis, Philadelphia.
Wertz, F.J. (1986) 'The question of the reliability of psychological research', *Journal of Phenomenological Psychology*, **17** (2) 181–205.

What You Need to Read

This should include the following:

Bryman, A. (1988) *Quantity and Quality in Social Research*, Unwin Hyman, London.
Darling, V.H. and Rogers, J. (1986) *Research for Practising Nurses*, Macmillan, Basingstoke.
Long, A.F. (1984) *Research into Health and Illness: Issues in Design, Analysis and Practice*, Gower, Aldershot.
Watson, J. (1985) *Nursing: Human Science and Human Care: A Theory of Nursing*, Appleton-Century-Crofts, Connecticut.

Sampling Methods

The purpose of research is usually to explore various themes and trends throughout a certain population of people (e.g. all the nurses in the UK or all the nurses working in medical wards in a group of hospitals). It is usually impractical to attempt to collect date from every member of that population. Therefore it is necessary to choose a sample from that population. A sample is a group of people from a larger population (although a sample may also be a collection of records, a number of observations and so on). It is usual to try to select a sample of people that is representative of the larger group. There are various ways of selecting a sample.

You will need to consider some of the following different methods of sampling:

- Simple random sampling
- Stratified random sampling
- Cluster sampling
- Opportunistic sample
- Quota sampling

- Convenience sampling
- Strategic informant sampling
- Purposive sampling
- Snowball sampling

You may find the following references useful when considering how to select a sample:

- Field, P.A. and Morse, J.M. (1985) *Nursing Research: The Application of Qualitative Approaches*, Croom Helm, London.
- Reid, N.G. and Boore, J.R.P. (1987) *Research Methods and Statistics in Health Care*, Arnold, London.
- Smith, H.W. (1981) *Strategies of Social Research: The Methodological Imagination*, 2nd edn, Prentice-Hall, Englewood Cliffs, New Jersey.

The sample that you need for your study will be determined to a large degree by what you are researching, what methods you are using and the time you have available. You need to discuss the question of sampling with your tutor or lecturer.

6.1 Structured Interviews

You will need to know the following:

- What a structured interview is;
- The difference between a structured interview and an unstructured interview;
- How to analyse a structured interview;
- The limitations of the use of structured interviews.

Structured Interviews

A structured interview uses an *interview schedule* which, in its strongest form, is like a *questionnaire*. The researcher uses a list of set questions which he or she asks of every person that he or she interviews. This interview schedule is designed and piloted well before the main interviews take place and is designed to cover everything that the researcher wants to find out from his or her respondents. One of the advantages of this approach is that it allows the researcher to organise and analyse his or her findings relatively easily. After the interviews, he or she can draw together all of the responses to the first question, all the responses to the second and so on. On the other hand, the structured interview allows no scope for *in-depth* interviewing. The interviewer cannot follow up subsequent questions that occur to him or her, nor can he or she follow 'hunches' and ask the respondent to elaborate on particular issues. This is particularly important if the researcher also wants to find out *why* people feel the way they do: the structured interview tends not to access this sort of information.

The structured interview cannot, by its design, cope with the spontaneous responses that people make nor the off-the-cuff impressions that respondents may want to offer. On the other hand, it can offer an economical way of gathering a lot of useful information quickly. The *depth* of the interview is largely determined by the *nature of the research questions* and the *level of understanding required by the researcher*.

An alternative to the completely structured interview is the *semi-structured* one. In the semi-structured interview, the researcher has a number of fixed questions prepared beforehand but he or she also builds in scope to ask *subsequent* questions, should the need arises. This breaks up the strict format of the structured approach and can yield 'richer' data. As well as obtaining *quantitative* data (from the structured part of the interview) the researcher also obtains more *qualitative* data (in the form of opinions, explanations and personal accounts). On the other hand, the data that arise out of these interviews can be more difficult to analyse because of the fact that the structure has been loosened.

Unstructured Interviews

The unstructured interview takes a very different approach to data collection. Usually, the researcher has some idea of the area on which he or she wants to focus the interview but, after that, the researcher remains open to whatever the respondent wants to say about that area of study. In this style of interviewing, the *respondent* has much more control over how the interview proceeds. The researcher can have little idea, beforehand, what *sort* of interview he or she will be conducting, nor can he or she know in advance what sorts of things the respondent will talk about. The net result of all this is that the researcher is likely to be faced with a wide range of different sorts of personal accounts that require analysis. Necessarily, the analysis of unstructured interviews is different to the analysis of structured ones. Various analysis methods have been devised to cope with the varied nature of the information gleaned from unstructured interviews. Some of these include the following:

• Content analysis
• Phenomenological analysis
• Grounded theory
• Ethnographic analysis.

If you are thinking about using the unstructured approach to interviews, you *must* know, beforehand, how you will analyse the interview transcripts. This is, of course, true, of *all* data collection methods: you must know, before you collect your data, how you will analyse it.

The following points should be borne in mind when using unstructured interviews:

- They are very time consuming: an interview may last half and hour or it may run for a number of hours.
- They should be taped – you cannot expect to remember the details of what was said in an interview if you rely on taking notes.
- The tapes should be *transcribed*. That is to say that all the words that are spoken by both the interviewer and the respondent should be written or typed out afterwards. There is some debate about whether or not this *always* has to happen. Some writers have suggested that you can work directly from the tapes. We suggest that you only use this approach once you have had considerable experience of working with unstructured interview.
- Whatever method of analysis you use, you must be clear about both the theoretical and *procedural* approaches that are to be adopted. Phenomenological and grounded theory approaches, for example, are based on highly complex philosophical ideas about the nature of knowledge and about ways of doing research. If you want to use these approaches, you need to know about these things. If not, you will be safer using a form of simple *content analysis*. There has been a tendency, in recent years, for some nurse researchers to use terms such as 'phenomenological' and 'hermeneutic' in fairly loose ways, and others have claimed that their studies involved 'modified grounded theory'. Theoretical clarity is essential in these matters – particularly in the qualitative field.

Further Reading

Burnard, P. (1992) 'Some problems in understanding other people: analysing talk in research, counselling and psychotherapy', *Nurse Education Today*, **12**, 130–6.

Kleinman, A. (1988) *The Illness Narratives: Suffering, Healing and the Human Condition*, Basic Books, New York.

Lofland, J. and Lofland, L.H. (1984) *Analysing Social Settings: A Guide to Qualitative Observation and Analysis*, Wadsworth, Belmont, California.

Morrison, P. (1992) *Professional Caring in Practice: A Psychological Analysis*, Avebury, Aldershot.

Strauss, A.L. (1987) *Qualitative Analysis for Social Scientists*, Cambridge University Press, Cambridge.

Turner, B. (1981) 'Some practical aspects of qualitative data analysis: one way of organising the cognitive processes associated with the generation of grounded theory', *Quality and Quantity*, **15**, 225–47.

Exercise 6.1

Aim of the exercise: To explore the use of the unstructured interview.

Planning stage: This activity needs to be carried out with one other person: a colleague or a friend. Allow yourself plenty of time to complete the exercise and make notes of what you do, as you go.

Equipment required: Notebook, pen and access to a nursing library; tape recorder.

What to do: Ask a friend to give you ten minutes of their time. In that ten minutes and without prior preparation, ask them to tell you about their work. Encourage the flow of conversation by asking any questions that come to mind and which have a bearing on the topic. Make notes about your colleague's responses or make a tape recording of the interview. If you can, repeat the process with one other friend.

Evaluation: When you have completed the interview(s), ask yourself the following questions about the data you have in front of you:

• Does it represent a detailed account of the colleague's work?
• Did the conversation 'flow' in an orderly manner and have a beginning, a middle and an end?
• How much did I talk during the interview?
• To what degree did I influence the sort of answers that the colleague offered?
• If two people were interviewed, was the content of both interviews similar in depth and breadth?
• Could I have collected the data more effectively?
• What sort of problems will I have in analysing these data?

As another level of evaluation, it is useful, before you finish the activity, to note down:

(a) what you learned from doing the activity,
(b) how you will use what you learned,
(c) how what you have learned relates to what you have read, and
(d) what you need to learn next.

You have conducted an unstructured interview. Such an approach may be useful in certain circumstances and we will return to this issue further on in this chapter. The structured interview offers alternative method of collecting information about a topic. As you work through the next exercise, consider the advantages and disadvantages of the structured approach to interviewing. The structured interview is distinguished by at least the following criteria:

- There are a limited number of questions.
- These questions have a specified number of possible answers.
- The answers are easier to quantify that the answers identified by the un-structured approach.
- The researcher specifies the questions to be asked.

Exercise 6.2

Aim of the exercise: to devise a short structured interview schedule and to use this as a basis for carrying out an interview.

Planning stage: This activity needs to be carried out with one other person – a colleague or a friend. Allow yourself plenty of time to complete the exercise and make notes of what you do, as you go.

Equipment / resources required: Notebook, pen and access to a nursing library.

What to do: Write out ten questions that you would like to ask someone about their job (see the section headed 'Open and Closed Questions', below, about different sorts of questions). Then ask those questions of your colleague and note down his answers. If possible, repeat the process with one or more colleagues.

Evaluation: Look at the responses that you elicited from your colleague(s) and ask yourself the following questions:

- Did I find out what I wanted to find out?
- Did my questions elicit the sort of answers that I anticipated that they would?
- How will I analyse the answers that I was offered?
- How could I improve my interview schedule?

If you can, discuss your questions and your colleague(s) responses with someone who has used a structure interview approach in his own research. Develop with you colleagues a list of the pros and cons of the unstructured and structured approaches to interviewing. Discuss when the unstructured and the structured approaches may be used to advantage.

As another level of evaluation, it is useful, before you finish the activity, to note down:

(a) what you learned from doing the activity,
(b) how you will use what you learned,
(c) how what you have learned relates to what you have read, and
(d) what you need to learn next.

Interviews used in research need not be of an entirely unstructured or an entirely structured nature. Many research reports combine both styles to very good effect. Now read the following papers about interviewing:

Hagan, T. (1986) 'Interviewing the downtrodden' in Ashworth, P., Giorgi, A. and de Koning, A. J.J. (eds) *Qualitative Research in Psychology*, Duquesne University Press, Pittsburgh, Pennsylvania, pp. 332–60.
Oppenheim, A.N. (1992) *Questionnaire Design, Interviewing and Attitude Measurement*, 2nd edn, Pinter, London.

Open and Closed Questions

Two types of questions may be described. Closed questions are those that elicit a restricted range of answers (in extreme, these answers may be 'yes' or 'no'). In some cases, the interviewer offers the respondent the range of possible answers. Examples of closed questions are:

• Do you smoke? Yes? No?
• How satisfied are you with your present state of health? Very satisfied? Satisfied? Uncertain? Dissatisfied? Very satisfied?

Open questions are those that elicit answers which the interviewer cannot anticipate and are usually lengthier and more divergent than the answers to closed questions. Open questions usually begin with the words: what, why, where or how? Examples of open questions are:

• What are your views on smoking?
• Why are you dissatisfied with your health?

Both closed and open questions may be used in research interviews. Methods of analysing the data obtained from the two types of question may differ.

Structured interviews that use closed questions may be analysed *quantitatively*. Unstructured interviews that use open questions may be analysed *qualitatively*. In between these two extremes are semi-structured interviews that may combine open and closed questions about the same topic. These semi-structured interviews may be analysed using both quantitative and/or qualitative methods.

6.2 Questionnaires

Simply stated, the questionnaire differs only from the structured interview by the degree of personal involvement on the part of the researcher at the point of data collection.

You will need to know the following:

- What a questionnaire is;
- What types of questionnaire there are;
- What are the advantages and disadvantages of questionnaires.

Two Types of Questionnaire

There are at least two major types of questionnaires: those that attempt to measure the structure and strength of attitudes and those that gather information about things. The attitudinal questionnaire consists of a series of questions that check people's opinions about events, situations, people and/or concepts. An attitudinal questionnaire, might, for example, try to identify people's attitudes towards mentally ill people being looked after in the community or patients' satisfaction levels with regard to their care in hospital. Attitudinal questions tend to focus on how people *think, feel* or *behave* with regard to the topic under consideration. Attitudinal questionnaires can often result in an overall *score*. This scoring mechanism usually operates on the basis that a *low* score relates to a *negative* attitude while a *high* score relates to a *positive* attitude.

A common method of collecting attitudinal data from a questionnaire is the inclusion of *Likert-type* items (named after the psychologist, Rene Likert). Figure 6.1 shows an example of such an item. Study the characteristics of it, try to read Likert's original paper (see Further reading, below) and then consult other books about the details of constructing such items.

Questionnaires that gather information about things do just that: they ask the respondent to report particular and specific information by ticking boxes or by answering specific questions – often in a 'yes/no' format. These sorts of questionnaires cannot be *scored*. Instead, the information that is gathered

	Strongly agree	Agree	Undecided	Disagree	Strongly disagree	Please leave blank
I get paid enough for the job I do						

Figure 6.1

from them can be illustrated in a series of tables. An example of an information-seeking questionnaire might be one that asks respondents about their nurse education, previous work experience and current job. The information that was gleaned from such a questionnaire might include the respondents' ages, sex, qualifications, training experiences and so forth.

Some questionnaires combine *both* forms of information gathering. It is important, however, to be clear about *which* questions are of an 'attitudinal' type and which are of an 'information gathering' type. This combination technique can allow the research to explore relationships (or lack of them) between concrete information and views and opinions. The researcher might, for example, want to explore whether or not there were differences in perceptions about mentally ill people between *psychiatric* nurses and *general* nurses. To do this, the researcher would have to collect some information about the nurses' background *as well* as asking them about their attitudes.

Further Reading

Anthonak, R.F. and Livneh, H. (1988) *The Measurement of Attitudes towards People with Disabilities: Methods, Psychometrics and Scales*, Charles C. Thomas, Springfield, Illinois.
Likert, R. (1932) 'A technique for the measurement of attitudes', *Archives of Psychology*, **140**, 1–55.
Sommer, B. and Sommer, R. (1991) *A Practical Guide to Behavioural Research: Tools and Techniques*, 3rd edn, Oxford University Press, Oxford.

Questionnaire Construction

Designing questionnaires is not easy. Oppenheim, in the preface to his classic book on questionnaire design, had this to say:

83

The world is full of well-meaning people who believe that anyone who can write plain English and has a modicum of common sense can produce a good questionnaire. This book is not for them (Oppenheim, 1992).

As a rule, if there is a ready-made questionnaire to hand, that has been properly tested for validity and reliability and which you do not have to modify, then you are best advised to use that. If you *have* or want to design a questionnaire, May (1993) suggests the following stages:

1. What is the aim of the research?
2. What information is required to fulfil these aims?
3. Undertake preliminary reading around the topic and initial fieldwork.
4. What type of questionnaire will be used and how will the sample be derived?
5. Consider the most appropriate questions to ask, which will depend upon the aims of the research, the target group and the time and resources at your disposal.
6. Construct a first draft, taking into account that pre-coded questions are easier to analyse and the order of question is the best social-psychological sequence.
7. Pilot the questionnaire and elicit the opinions of the sub-sample, gain critical but supportive comments from those familiar with the design and analysis of questionnaires.
8. Edit the questionnaire to check on form, content and sequence of questions, make sure the questionnaire is neatly typed and all instructions and coding are clear and filter questions, if any, are understandable.
9. Administer the questionnaire, noting the dynamics for the interviews and comments of the interviewers (if used).
10. Analyse the questionnaire drawing upon statistical techniques.

Exercise 6.3

Aim of the exercise: To become familiar with various types of questionnaires

Planning stage: The exercise can be carried out alone or with a group of colleagues. Allow yourself plenty of time to complete the exercise and make notes of what you do, as you go. If you work with friends or colleagues, decide whether you will carry out similar tasks or you will divide up the work between you.

Equipment required: Notebook, pen and access to a nursing library.

What to do: Sit down and draw up a short questionnaire of six questions. The questions should be designed to answer one of the following research questions:

- Is nursing stressful?
- Are some nurses more assertive than others?
- Do nurses use a nursing model in their practice?

Do no prior reading before attempting this part of the exercise.
    When you have written your six questions, go to the library and find the following books.

Converse, J.M. and Presser, S. (1986) *Survey Questions: Hand-crafting the Standardized Questionnaire*, Sage, Beverly Hills.
Sudman, S. and Bradburn, N.M. (1987) *Asking Questions: A Practical Guide to Questionnaire Design*, Jossey Bass, San Francisco.

Read through the sections of questionnaires and answer the following questions:

- What is a questionnaire?
- What is a questionnaire for?
- What distinguishes a questionnaire from an interview?
- How may questionnaire data analysed?
- What principles go into the production of questionnaires?

Now read through your own questions and see to what degree they need to be modified. Then try to modify them in the light of your reading.

Evaluation: Try out your modified questionnaire on a friend. Ask her to act as 'devil's advocate' and raise any objections she may have about the construction of your short questionnaire. Try, also, to show the questionnaire to a tutor or to someone with research experience and ask their opinion of your work.
    If you worked in a group, share your experiences and note the degree to which problems in questionnaire construction were common to a number of the group members.
    As another level of evaluation, it is useful, before you finish the activity, to note down:

(a) what you learned from doing the activity,
(b) how you will use what you learned,
(c) how what you have learned relates to what you have read, and
(d) what you need to learn next.

Advantages and Disadvantages of Questionnaires

Advantages

- Questionnaires offer a fairly straightforward way of collecting data, quickly and efficiently.
- They are cheap to use.
- They can enable the researcher to collect information anonymously.
- They are usually easy to analyse.
- Large batches of data can be collected with them.

Disadvantages

- The researcher has no personal contact with the respondent.
- They can be difficult to construct.
- They involve 'forced choice' of response from the respondent.

Try to add to both of these lists, from your reading on the topic.

6.3 Experiments

Experiments are systematic attempts to test out a theory (usually stated in the form of a hypothesis). Experimental research tries to identify causal relationships between variables, and tries to establish 'laws'. It is not anticipated that many nurses coming fresh to research will be planning experimental studies. It is usefull, however, to be able to read experimental research studies both for their content and also to be critical of them.

You will need to know the following:

- What a hypothesis is;
- Some of the terms associated with experimental research;
- How to become critical of experimental research reports.

Exercise 6.4

Aim of the exercise: To explore the notions of hypothesis and null hypothesis.

Planning stage: This activity can be carried out by the person working on her own or by a group of people. Allow yourself plenty of time to complete the exercise and make notes of what you do, as you go. If you work with friends or colleagues, decide whether you will carry out similar tasks or whether you will divide up the work between you.

Equipment required: Notebook, pen and access to a nursing library; tape recorder.

What to do: Go to the library and find the following books. Read through the sections on hypotheses. These are identified by page numbers following the references:

Dixon, B.R., Bouma, G.D. and Atkinson, G.B.J. (1987) *A Handbook of Social Science Research*, Oxford University Press, Oxford, pp. 53–8.
Leedy, P.D. (1985) *Practical Research: Planning and Design*, 3rd edn, Macmillan, New York, pp. 5–6, 64–5.

Evaluation: Ask yourself the following questions:

• What is a hypothesis?
• What is a null hypothesis?
• How do you use a hypothesis?
• What is the difference between a hypothesis and an assumption?
• What does the term 'variable' mean?

Now talk to your tutor about the concept of a hypothesis.
    As another level of evaluation, it is useful, before you finish the activity, to note down:

(a) what you learned from doing the activity,
(b) how you will use what you learned,
(c) how what you have learned relates to what you have read, and
(d) what you need to learn next.

Issues in Using Experiments

It is unlikely, in a small-scale research project, that you will design and execute a social science experiment. However, it is important that you know something about the nature and design of such experiments. Why? Because experiments formed the basis of the knowledge base in the biological sciences and to a lesser extent, the social sciences. Here are some of the terms and concepts that you should become familiar with and that are related to experimental design:

- Experimental design seeks to establish *causal* relationships. That is to say that they don't just describe things but they seek to *explain* them by establishing *causes* for things. If you are able to find a *cause* for things, you are in a better position to *predict* future events. However, all this hangs on a particular view of science and the idea of establishing causal relationships in human research is very difficult.
- In an experiment, the researcher tries to establish almost total control over the conditions in which things occur. In order to be able to do this, he or she must first identify a concisely worded *hypothesis*: a statement that he or she seeks to prove or disprove. It should be noted that it is not normally necessary (though sometimes a chosen path) to develop a hypothesis in *other* sorts of research. Normally, hypotheses are only associated with experimental research.
- Often, in experiments, at least two groups are employed: an *experimental* group and a *control* group. The experimental group is exposed to the experimental treatment while the control group is not. Both groups are matched for similarity in all important respects – for example, sex, age, social class. In this way, the researcher can study what differences, if any, the new treatment makes. All the time he or she is studying the experimental group he or she can check what is happening to the 'untreated' or control group. If changes *do* occur in the experimental group, it can more easily be demonstrated that the change occurred *because of* the new treatment. Constant comparison between the two groups allows for more rigorous hypothesis testing.
- The above scenario spells out the *ideal* situation. Real life is often more complicated and even a laboratory experiment can be *contaminated* in many ways. Good researchers are loath to draw firm conclusions from their findings until they have been able to reproduce very similar experimental conditions over and over again. Even then, the question of causality is open to question and this is a debate that has raged for many years in the research literature.
- Most frequently, experiments are carried out under laboratory conditions. If they are done in 'real life' settings, it becomes much more difficult to design and execute a controlled experiment.

Robson summarises the characteristics of experiments as follows:

- The assignment of subjects to different conditions;
- The manipulation of one or more variables (called independent variables) by the researcher;
- The measurement of the effects of this manipulation on one or more other variables (called dependent variables);
- The control of all other variables (Robson, 1993).

Further Reading

Dickson, J. (1984) 'Effects of nursing intervention on nutritional and performance status in cancer patients', *Nursing Research*, **33** (6) 330–5.

Mitchell, J. and Jolley, J. (1985) *Research Design Explained*, Holt, Rinehart & Winston, New York.

Polit, D. and Hungler, B. (1987) *Nursing Research: Principles and Methods*, 3rd edn, Lippincott, Philadelphia.

Rice, V. and Johnson, J. (1984) 'Pre-admission self instruction booklets, post admission exercise performance and teaching time', *Nursing Research*, **33** (3) 147–51.

Robson, C. (1983) *Experiment, Design and Statistics in Psychology*, 2nd edn, Penguin, Harmondsworth.

Exercise 6.5

Aim of the exercise: To explore some of the terms commonly used in experimental research.

Planning stage: This activity can be carried out by the person working on her own or by a group of people. Allow yourself plenty of time to complete the exercise and make notes of what you do, as you go. If you work with friends or colleagues, decide whether you will carry out similar tasks or whether you will divide up the work between you.

Equipment required: Notebook, pen and access to a nursing library.

What to do: Go to the library and study books on research and devise definitions for the following terms. You will find an extensive list of such books in the back of this one. Make notes of your definitions.

• Control group
• Experimental group
• Statistical significance
• Sampling
• Confounding variables

Now read the following two research reports and note how these terms are used. In coming to terms with the concepts involved in the use of these words, you are beginning to get to grips with the concepts involved in doing experimental work. As you read these reports, try to evaluate the degree to which the writers have addressed problems presented by these concepts.

Luker, K.A. (1982) *Evaluating Health Visiting Practice*, RCN, London.
Hayward, J. (1975) *Information: A Prescription Against Pain*, RCN, London.

Evaluation: Discuss the above terms with friends and with a tutor and make sure that you are clear about their use.

As another level of evaluation, it is useful, before you finish the activity, to note down:

(a) what you learned from doing the activity,
(b) how you will use what you learned,
(c) how what you have learned relates to what you have read, and
(d) what you need to learn next.

6.4 Observation

By the end of this section you will have discovered:

- What sort of information is being sought through observation;
- Some of the problems associated with observation;
- What types of observational methods can be used.

Exercise 6.6

Aim of the exercise: To explore problems and practical issues associated with observation

Planning stage: You can do this exercise on your own or in the company of a small group of colleagues, friends or students. Allow yourself plenty of time to complete the exercise and make notes of what you do, as you go. If you work with friends or colleagues, decide whether you will carry out similar tasks or whether you will divide up the work between you.

Equipment required: Notebook, pen and access to a nursing library.

What to do:

Stage One:
Go to somewhere crowded or busy (e.g. a bus station, an out-patients department, a staff cafeteria. Sit and observe people for about ten minutes. Make notes about your observations.
Now consider the following questions:

- What sort of things did you observe?
- How did you decide on what to observe and what to ignore?
- How did you make notes on what you observed?
- Did you try to interpret what people were doing and why they were doing it?

In considering these issues you are beginning to appreciate the difficulties that all researchers face when trying to decide on how to collect data by means of observation.
Some researchers have found it useful to use a system for recording what they see.

Stage Two:
First, identify in your own mind what it is you want to observe when you go to the crowded place, identified above. You might, for instance, be interested in how many people get on a particular bus when it stops at a bus station, or you might want to observe how many people choose salad as a meal in the staff cafeteria. What you can never do is observe everything that is going on in any given situation. You must decide what is important for your project. You must also try to refrain from interpreting what you see. You are not there to make assumptions about people's behaviour, you are there to observe and record. At a later stage you may want to ask people why they did things but that comes later.
To aid your observation, draw up a simple checklist or grid to help you record what you see. Now go back to the crowded place for a further ten minutes and use your checklist and observe again.
Now ask yourself the following questions:

- Was the second stage of the exercise easier or more difficult than the first?
- In what ways did your checklist help or hinder you?
- Did your checklist work?

In these two activities you have explored some of the problems associated with observation in research. Now read the following to clarify further how observational methods may be used to collect research data. Read, too, the section below on 'Aspects of Observation in Research'.

Henerson, M.E., Morris, L.L. and Fitz-Gibbon, C.T. (1987) *How to Measure Attitudes*, Sage, Beverly Hills, ch. 9.

Lofland, J. and Lofland, L. (1984) *Analysing Social Settings*, 2nd edn, Wadsworth, Newark, New Jersey.

Taylor, S. and Bogdan, R. (1984) *Introduction to Qualitative Research Methods*, 2nd edn, Wiley, New York.

Aspects of Observation in Research

Two Types of Observational Method

1. *Non-Participant Observation*: Here, the researcher enters a social setting as an observer and sits and records examples of behaviour or action that he is researching. He does not attempt to influence the situation that he is in and does not attempt to stop anything from happening. On the other hand, of course, the very presence of the researcher may change what is happening. This has been called the 'Hawthorne Effect' (Tajfel and Fraser, 1978).
2. *Participant Observation*: Here, the researcher enters a social situation and works alongside the people in that situation, thus fulfilling a dual role (*a*) as a worker and (*b*) as an observer.

You may want to consider the pros and cons of these two approaches, whether or not there are ethical problems with either approach and the appropriateness of either method in answering a particular research question.

Sommer and Sommer offer the following list of steps for systematic observation:

1. Specify the question(s) of interest (reason for doing the study).
2. Do casual observation, distinguishing between observation (the actual behaviour seen) and inference (interpretation, what you think it means).
3. Are the observational categories clearly described?
4. Design the measurement instruments (i.e. checklists, categories, coding systems, etc.).
5. Is the study designed so that it will be *valid* (i.e. does it measure what it is supposed to measure and have some generalisability)?
6. Train observers in the use of the instruments.
7. *Do a pilot test.*

(*a*) Test the actual observation procedure;

(*b*) Check reliability of the categories using at least two independent observers.

8. Review procedure and instruments in the light of the pilot test results. If substantial changes are made, run another pilot test.
9. Collect data.
10. Compile, analyse and interpret results (Sommer and Sommer, 1991).

Further Reading

Becker, H.S. and Geer, B. (1992) 'Participant observation: the analysis of qualitative field data' in R.G. Burgess (ed.) *Field Research: A Sourcebook and Field Manual*, Allen & Unwin, London.

Jorgenson, D.L. (1989) *Participant Observation*, Sage, London.

Kirk, J. and Miller, M.L. (1986) *Reliability and Validity in Qualitative Research*, Sage, London.

Robertson, C.M. (1982) 'A Description of Participant Observation of Clinical Teaching', *Journal of Advanced Nursing*, **7** (6) 549–54.

Conclusion

In this chapter we have considered four main types of data collection methods. If you can become familiar with the main skills involved in each of these you will be better able to examine, critically, the research literature.

You may find, however, that these methods are not the ones best suited to addressing your own research project. In the next chapter, we consider some other methods, other than the more traditional, which may offer more scope or variety.

Learning Check

If You are Working on Your Own

Read through the notes that you have kept whilst completing the exercises in this chapter and consider the following questions:

• What new knowledge have I gained?
• What new skills have I developed?
• How has my thinking about research changed?
• What do I need to do now?

Check that you have made reference cards for any new references that you have found whilst working on the exercises in this chapter.

If You are Working in a Small Group

Pair off and nominate one of you as A and one of you as B. For five minutes, A talks to B about what she has learned and B listens. This should *not* be a conversation: B's only role is to listen. After five minutes, roles are reversed and B talks to A about what she has learned and A listens. After the second five minutes, re-form into a group a discuss the experience.

If You are a Tutor and/or Facilitator

- Use the above pairs exercise with the group you are working with.
- Hold two 'rounds' in which each person in turn says *(a)* what she liked least about doing the activities and *(b)* what she liked most about doing the activities.

7

Other Methods of Collecting Data

Aims of this Chapter

These are:

- To explore a variety of other research data collection methods;
- To consider the appropriateness or otherwise of these methods for your project;
- To identify key references for further reading on these methods.

Introduction

In the last chapter we considered four methods of collecting data: interviews, questionnaires, experiments and observation. We noted that these were perhaps the most frequently used methods in many social science research projects, including those carried out in nursing. In this chapter we examine some other methods that you may want to consider for your project or which you may come across in your search and examination of the literature and previous research. As we have noted, there is no right or wrong way of collecting data. Different projects, different research questions and different levels of experience will influence the decision to choose one method rather than another. Appropriate choice of method is the key to success in research and arguably it is useful to have an informed awareness of a wide range of such methods.

The methods we consider in this chapter are:

- use of existing records
- repertory grid technique
- critical incident technique
- multiple sort technique
- use of existing scales, inventories, tests and assessment tools
- semantic differential.

It is not claimed that this is an exhaustive list of all possible data collection techniques and you are advised to be on the look out for other methods not covered in this book.

What You Need to Read

This should include the following:

Field, P.A. and Morse, J.M. (1985) *Nursing Research: The Application of Qualitative Approaches*, Croom Helm, London.
Sweener, M.A. and Oliveri, P. (1981) *An Introduction to Nursing Research: Research, Measurement and Computers in Nursing*, Lippincott, Philadelphia.
Van Maanen, J. (1983) *Qualitative Methodology*, Sage, Beverly Hills, California.
Verhonick, P. and Seaman, C. (1978) *Research Methods for Undergraduate Students in Nursing*, Appleton-Century-Crofts, New York.

7.1 Use of Existing Records

By the end of this section you will have discovered:

- What sort of records can be used in a research project;
- How to gain access to records;
- How to use records in research.

Sources of Existing Data

It is sometimes thought that a researcher must collect new data. An alternative view is that it can be extremely informative to explore existing datasets. These can often lead to researchers asking new and important questions, or can shed light on 'real world' problems, without the need to design and execute large-scale studies. There are often huge datasets sitting waiting to be re-examined. Here are some of the sources of such datasets:

- Lists of accidents and incidents occurring in clinical areas;
- In psychiatric units, records of disturbed behaviour and of seclusion;
- Existing datasets collected by other colleagues and friends during other research projects;
- Shift work listings, off-duty rosters, workload patterns and other management records;

- *Social Trends* published by HMSO.
- Published sets of data (e.g. those published by the Economic and Social Research Council (ESRC) Data Archive). This organisation offers the possibility of purchasing at nominal cost huge sets of data collected on various topics throughout the world. The data arrives in a 'raw' state and computing and statistical knowledge is required to make use of such datasets.

Further Reading

Harris, R.B. and Hyman, R.B. (1984) 'Clean versus sterile tracheostomy care and level of pulmonary infection', *Nursing Research*, **33** (2) 80–5.
While, A.E. (1987) 'Records as a data source: the case for health-visitor records', *Journal of Advanced Nursing*, **12** (6) 757–63.

Exercise 7.1

Aim of the exercise: To explore the use of collecting data from a set of existing records.

Planning stage: This exercise can be carried out by a person working on her own or in a small group. Allow yourself plenty of time to complete the exercise and make notes of what you do, as you go. If you work with friends or colleagues, decide whether you will all carry out similar tasks or whether you will divide up the work between you.

Equipment required: Notebook, pen and access to a nursing library.

What to do: Ask a senior nurse if you may have access to one of the following sets of records. Be sure to state why you want to look at them and tell her that you will destroy your written work after you have completed the exercise.

- Off-duty sheets for the past month;
- The accident book on your ward;
- Ward report sheets for the past month.

Sit down with a set of records and note the types of information that are contained on these records. For example, off-duty sheets may contain information about:

- How many qualified and unqualified staff have been on and off duty;

- The numbers of staff nurses on duty per day, per shift, per week, etc.

The accident book may contain information about:

- The time that accidents occur;
- The age of the persons involved;
- The location of accidents.

The ward report sheets may contain information about:

- The number of staff on duty and off sick on a particular day;
- The number of patients on the ward on a particular day;
- Any new admissions and any discharges to and from the ward.

Devise a simple method of collecting *some* of that information onto one sheet. Then look through the data that you have collected and see if any particular *patterns* occur within those data. For example, if you are considering the staff off-duty sheet, you could ask the following questions in order to establish trends or patterns:

- Are there particular days when the ward is poorly staffed and does this fact coincide with work requirements or other factors?
- Are there more trained staff on duty on some days and, if so, why may this be the case?
- How are any part-time staff allocated shifts? Is this allocation running to a fixed pattern or does it vary from week to week?

Gradually, you will be able to develop a picture from the data that will tell you a considerable amount about the ward and the way the ward works. This picture will be considerably more detailed *after* you have filtered out certain trends and patterns than was the case before you sat down with the records.

This approach to working with records can lead you to ask other questions about the topic that you are interested in and can point your research in other, more useful, directions that may not have been at first apparent.

Evaluation: Discuss your findings in your small group and see to what degree there is agreement about trends and patterns emerging out of the data.

As another level of evaluation, it is useful, before you finish the activity, to note down:

(a) what you learned from doing the activity,
(b) how you will use what you learned,
(c) how what you have learned relates to what you have read, and
(d) what you need to learn next.

Remember to destroy all your notes after use. Not to do so is to contravene the Data Protection Act 1985 and is to breach confidentiality.

7.2   Repertory Grid Technique

By the end of this section you will have discovered:

• Whether or not Kelly's repertory grid technique may be usefully considered for your own research project.

Personal Construct Theory and Repertory Grids

The repertory grid technique is based on Kelly's (1955) personal construct theory. In its simplest form it seeks to identify the characteristics that an individual looks for in other people and in the world around him. These characteristics, Kelly calls 'constructs' and he argues that they are usually bipolar or two-sided in nature. Thus the person who sees some people as 'caring' by nature, will tend to compare those people to others that they see as being 'uncaring'. Kelly also argued that each person's set of ways of seeing other things or people (her 'constructs'), varied from person to person.

Kelly used the word 'element' to describe events, things, people that are being viewed by the person through her construct system. Thus it is possible to consider three elements: *(a)* a friend, *(b)* a doctor and *(c)* a nurse. It is then possible to consider in what ways *two* of those elements are similar and different from the third. For example, you may consider that the doctor and the nurse are both PROFESSIONALS and the friend is NOT PROFESSIONAL. Alternatively, you may consider that the nurse and the friend are both APPROACHABLE and the doctor is DISTANT. In these examples, then, the friend, doctor and nurse are ELEMENTS and the descriptions PROFESSIONAL–NOT PROFESSIONAL and APPROACHABLE–DISTANT are both bipolar CONSTRUCTS.

This approach to identifying people's characteristic ways of viewing people and the world around them can be exploited for the purposes of research. The approach may be used to find out how a group of nurses perceive working in an accident and emergency unit or how they feel about their colleagues, their work, their training and so on. Much has been written about the personal construct approach and the use of the repertory grid technique in research, and the reader is referred to that for further information.

Further Reading

Bannister, D. and Fransella, F. (1986) *Inquiring Man*, 3rd edn, Croom Helm, London.

Beail, N. (1985) *Repertory Grid Technique and Personal Constructs*, Croom Helm, London.

Burnard, P. and Morrison, P. (1989) 'What is an interpersonally skilled person? A repertory grid account of professional nurses' views', *Nurse Education Today*, **9**, 384–91.

Morrison, P. (1990) 'An example of the use of repertory grid technique in assessing nurses' self-perceptions of caring', *Nurse Education Today*, **10**, 253–9.

Pollock, L.C. (1986) 'An introduction to the use of repertory grid technique as a research method and clinical tool for psychiatric nurses', *Journal of Advanced Nursing*, **11**, 439–45.

Stewart, V. and Stewart, A. (1981) *Business Applications of Repertory Grid*, McGraw-Hill, London.

Exercise 7.2

Aim of the exercise: To explore some basic principles of the repertory grid technique.

Planning stage: You can do this exercise on your own or in the company of a small group of colleagues, friends or students. Allow yourself plenty of time to complete the exercise and make notes of what you do, as you go. If you work with friends or colleagues, decide whether you will all carry out similar tasks or whether you will divide up the work between you.

Equipment required: Notebook, pen and access to a nursing library.

What to do: Consider the following list of types of people and put a name next to each:

1. A good friend
2. Your mother
3. Your father
4. A favourite teacher

5. Someone you don't like
6. Yourself.

This list is a list of 'elements' for you to consider.

Now think about those elements in threes, as listed below. Consider each of the three elements and identify the ways in which *two* of the people are similar and *different* from the third. In each case, write down the SIMILARITY and the DIFFERENCE in the space provided. This will produce a list of bipolar constructs and will offer you some ideas about how you, as an individual, tend to view people. It is notable that another person's list of constructs will be different from yours.

Three elements for comparison	Similarity	Difference
	(the emerging set of bipolar constructs)	
1, 2, 3		
4, 5, 6		
2, 3, 4		
1, 2, 6		
2, 5, 3		
3, 4, 6		

Now consider the range of personal constructs that have been elicited through this exercise. Are you surprised by the constructs or are they representative of the sorts of qualities that you imagined that you attributed to other people? Compare your findings with those of a colleague and identify the ways in which they are similar and different.

It is worth noting that there are numerous and sophisticated ways or processing the information obtained in this sort of way. For further details of the ways in which this is done, see the references to repertory grid techniques offered in the Further reading section, above.

Evaluation: If you are working in a small group, discuss your findings with your colleagues. Also, consider ways that you may use this approach in a research project.

As another level of evaluation, it is useful, before you finish the activity, to note down:

(a) what you learned from doing the activity,
(b) how you will use what you learned,

(c) how what you have learned relates to what you have read, and
(d) what you need to learn next.

7.3   Critical Incident Technique

By the end of this section you have discovered:

• How to consider using the critical incident technique.

Critical Incident Technique

Critical incident technique, in its simplest form, offers the opportunity to discover how people say they have reacted in certain situations. For example, it may be useful to find out how nursing assistants felt about how they acted in the event of a patient having a cardiac arrest. It may also be used to discover how different *groups* of people say they reacted in particular situations. For example, it may be interesting to find out how doctors, senior nurses *and* nursing assistants consider how they acted in the event of a patient having a cardiac arrest.

The critical incident technique is used to help people to reflect on past events and to note how they report their reactions to such events. Thus, a group of student nurses may be asked to describe how they dealt with their first experience of a patient having an epileptic fit.

Different methods of data collection may be used to gather examples of incidents for review and for identifying people's perceptions of those incidents. For example, the researcher may use interviews, questionnaires, records and self-report measures.

The analysis of the data obtained involves the classification of people's responses to incidents into particular categories. For example, ward sisters may be asked to think of a time when they were functioning particularly well in their role as teacher. The words and phrases that they use to describe their performance are then filtered into a variety of categories, e.g. 'effective communication', 'skilled behaviour', 'enjoyment' and so on. These categories can then be used to present the data in a written format and they may allow the researcher to offer answers to her research question.

Further Reading

Clamp, C.G.L. (1984) 'Learning Through Incidents: Studies in the Development and Use of Critical Incidents in the Teaching of Attitudes in Nursing', unpublished MPhil Thesis, University of London Institute of Education.

Cormack, D.F.S. (1983) *Psychiatric Nursing Described*, Churchill Livingstone, Edinburgh.

Cormack, D.F.S. (1984) 'Flanagan's Critical Incident Technique' in Cormack, D.F.S. (ed.) *The Research Process in Nursing*, Blackwell, Oxford, pp. 118–25.

Dunn, W.R. and Hamilton, D.D. (1986) 'The critical incident technique: a brief guide', *Medical Teacher*, **8** (3) 207–15.

Flanagan, J.C. (1954) 'The Critical Incident Technique', *Psychological Bulletin*, **51** (4) 327–58.

Exercise 7.3

Aim of the exercise: To explore one aspect of the critical incident technique.

Planning stage: You can do this exercise on your own or in the company of a small group of colleagues, friends or students. Allow yourself plenty of time to complete the exercise and make notes of what you do, as you go. If you work with friends or colleagues, decide whether you will all carry out similar tasks or you will divide the work between you.

Equipment required: Notebook, pen and access to a nursing library.

What to do: Consider one of the following incidents from your past:

• Observing patient having an epileptic fit;
• The fire alarm sounding when you were at work;
• Giving a patient an injection;
• Being present at a road traffic accident.

Now write down what happened and write down *what you did*. Now consider the following questions:

• Do you consider that your action was appropriate?
• If not, why not?
• How did you feel about what happened?
• In what ways could your performance have been improved?
• What did you learn from the incident?
• What would you do differently next time?

Now look through your responses and see whether or not certain trends occur and see whether or not those trends can be placed under certain broad headings.

Evaluation: If you are working in a small group, share experiences and reactions. Do your reactions fall into certain categories and can you agree, as a group, on the categories generated by this activity?

As another level of evaluation, it is useful, before you finish the activity, to note down:

(a) what you learned from doing the activity,
(b) how you will use what you learned,
(c) how what you have learned relates to what you have read, and
(d) what you need to learn next.

7.5 Multiple Sort Technique

By the end of this section you will have discovered:

• Whether or not the multiple sort technique may be suitable for your project.

The multiple sort method combines two other sorts of data collection methods: the 'Q' sort (Stephenson, 1953) and the repertory grid approach, described above. The exercise that follows explains the basic principles of the method.

Exercise 7.4

Aim of the exercise: To explore the use of the multiple sort technique.

Planning stage: This exercise involves two people: you, as the researcher, and a colleague as the informant. Allow yourself plenty of time to complete the exercise and makes notes, as you go.

Equipment required: Small pieces of paper or card, about 8 x 13 cm. Pencil and paper and access to a nursing library.

What to do: Write the following phrases onto separate cards:

PSYCHIATRIC NURSING   CARDIAC NURSING

GERIATRIC NURSING   MIDWIFERY

PAEDIATRIC NURSING   HEALTH VISITING

ORTHOPAEDIC NURSING	DISTRICT NURSING
OPHTHALMIC NURSING	MACMILLAN NURSING
ONCOLOGY NURSING	COMMUNITY PSYCHIATRIC NURSING
UROLOGICAL NURSING	
MENTAL HANDICAP NURSING	SCHOOL NURSING
	OCCUPATIONAL HEALTH NURSING
MEDICAL NURSING	
SURGICAL NURSING	INDUSTRIAL NURSING

Now ask your colleague to look through the cards and sort them into piles. The piles may represent any sort of differentiation at all. Your colleague is free to determine how she divides them up. Then ask your colleague to *Label* the piles that she has produced.

Make a note of the labels of the piles and the cards within each pile. Now have a go at sorting the cards yourself. See whether or not you produce a different set of piles and, perhaps, a different number of piles.

In doing this exercise you have been using the multiple sort technique: a technique that allows you to explore another person's viewpoint, style of differentiating between things and so forth.

Evaluation: Discuss the piles and their labels with your colleague and discuss ways that the method could be used in a research project.

As another level of evaluation, it is useful, before you finish the activity, to note down:

(a) what you learned from doing the activity,
(b) how you will use what you learned,
(c) how what you have learned relates to what you have read and
(d) what you need to learn next.

The Multiple Sorting Technique

The multiple sorting technique may be used for structuring an interview and collecting qualitative information. It has the distinct advantage of providing a structured interview format and statistical analysis procedure while at the same time it allows the informant to dictate what the important issues and considerations are. In so doing, it allows the researcher to gather rich details about the informant's views of the world which may be analysed both qualitatively and quantitatively.

The multiple sorting technique is a method which can be used to explore the important constructs which people use to structure and describe their experiences, by examining how they assign elements to conceptual categories. In effect, the multiple sorting technique allows the researcher to study individual perceptions of a specific research topic in a highly structured and organised manner.

Further Reading

Canter, D., Brown, J. and Groat, L. (1985) 'A multiple sorting procedure for studying conceptual systems' in Brenner, M., Brown, J. and Canter, D. (eds) *The Research Interview: Uses and Approaches*, Academic Press, London, pp. 79–114.

Groat, L. (1982) 'Meaning in post-modern architecture: an examination using the multiple sorting task', *Journal of Environmental Psychology*, **2** (3) 3–22.

Morrison, P. and Bauer, I. (1993) 'A clinical application of the clinical sorting technique', *International Journal of Nursing Studies,* **30** (6) 511–13.

Wilson, M.A. and Canter, D.V. (1990) 'The development of central concepts during professional education: a example of a multivariate model of the concept of architectural style', *Applied Psychology: an international review*, **39** (4) 431–55.

7.7 Use of Existing Scales, Inventories, Tests and Assessment Tools

By the end of this section you will have discovered:

- How to find existing scales, inventories, tests and assessment tools
- Whether or not such scales, inventories, tests or assessment tools would be useful in your research project.

Exercise 7.4

Aim of the exercise: To explore the use of pre-existing scales, inventories and assessment tools.

Planning stage: You can do this exercise on your own or in the company of a small group of colleagues, friends or students. Allow yourself plenty of time to complete the exercise and make notes of what you do, as you go. If you work with friends or colleagues, decide whether you will all carry out similar tasks or you will divide the work between you.

Equipment required: Notebook, pen and access to a nursing library.

What to do: Go to the library and locate one or more of the following sources of established scales, inventories, tests or assessment tools:

Anastasi, A. (1988) *Psychological Testing*, 6th edn, Macmillan, New York.
Antonak, R.F. and Livneh, H. (1988) *The Measurement of Attitudes toward People with Disabilities: Methods, Psychometrics and Scales*, Charles C. Thomas, Springfield, Illinois.
Bowling, A. (1991) *Measuring Health: A Review of Quality of Life Measurement Scales*, Open University Press, Milton Keynes.
Robinson, J.P. and Shaver, P.R. (1973) *Measurement of Social Psychological Attitudes*, Institute for Social Research, University of Michigan, Ann Arbor, Michigan.
Ward, M.J. and Felter, M.E. (1979) *Instruments for Use in Nursing Education Research*, Western Interstate Commission for Higher Education, Boulder, Colorado.

If you have difficulty in obtaining these particular items, consult the list of scales, inventories, tests and assessment tools in the compendium section at the back of this book.

Scan through the two of the instruments that you have found discussed in the literature and answer the following questions:

- How as the instrument developed?
- How was it tested?
- Does the instrument relate specifically to nursing? If not, could it be used in a nursing context?
- Does the instrument relate to a particular culture or does it claim to be applicable across a wide range of different cultures?
- Is it suitable for your particular needs? If not, why not?
- If you were to use it, would you need permission to use it?
- Could you analyse the data obtained?

Evaluation: Discuss your findings with a group of colleagues. If you find that you *do* want to use a particular instrument, discuss its use with a tutor first. You may be surprised at how many instruments have already been defined. Also, you may be able to adapt an existing instrument to suit your particular needs. If an a suitable instrument does exist, you may be advised to use it, rather than spend considerable time devising your own.

As another level of evaluation, it is useful, before you finish the activity, to note down:

(a) what you learned from doing the activity,
(b) how you will use what you learned,
(c) how what you have learned relates to what you have read, and
(d) what you need to learn next.

7.8 Semantic Differential

By the end of this section you will have discovered:

• What the semantic differential technique is;
• Whether or not you could use it in your research project.

Semantic Differential Technique

Semantic differential explores the ways that people use certain words to describe situations. It is a highly structured means of exploring people's perceptions of those situations, people or things. If we accept that each of us views a situation slightly differently and that when we describe a situation we each use different words in that description, then it may be useful to tap into the sets of words and meanings that various people use to describe things that they observe.

The semantic differential approach allows the researcher to explore the similarities and the differences between people's perceptions of situation, people and things. It is an underlying assumption of the technique that certain words mean the same sorts of things to various people.

The technique offers the subject a series of bipolar dimensions along which to rate themselves, other people or activities. For example, you may be asked to consider where you would place yourself, on the following dimension, in terms of caring. You can do this by placing a tick on the scale below:

caring| ....| ....| ....| ....| ....| ....|uncaring

Your rating along that dimension could then be compared with other people's ratings of themselves. Normally, you would be asked to rate yourself along a number of dimensions, and this way of working is explored in the exercise in the text.

Further Reading

Choon, G.L. And Skevington, S.M. (1984) 'How do women and men in nursing perceive each other?', in Skevington, S. (ed.), *Understanding Nurses*, Wiley, Chichester, pp. 101–11.
Kerlinger, F. (1986) *Foundations of Behavioural Research*, 3rd edn, CBS Publishing, Tokyo.
Osgood, C.E., Suci, G.J. and Tannenbaum, P.H. (1957) *The Measurement of Meaning*, University of Illinois Press, Urbana, Illinois.

Exercise 7.5

Aim of the exercise: To explore the use of the semantic differential approach.

Planning stage: This exercise is initially to be carried out by a person working on her own, yet in the company of others. In the evaluation stage, it is important that you work with a small group of colleagues. Allow yourself plenty of time to complete the exercise and make notes of what you do, as you go. If you work with friends or colleagues, decide whether you will all carry out similar tasks or you will divide the work between you.

Equipment required: Notebook, pen and access to a nursing library.

What to do: Consider the dimensions listed in Figure 7.1 and rate your own perception on the scale provided, by placing a tick at the appropriate points along the dimensions.

Your perceptions of an AIDS patient

AIDS patients may often be:

1. Weak							Powerful
2. Conformist							Non-conformist
3. Dominant							Submissive
4. Aggressive							Peaceful
5. Kind							Unkind
6. Logical							Intuitive
7. Stupid							Intelligent
8. Clean							Dirty
9. Happy							Sad
10. Moral							Immoral

Figure 7.1

Now draw a line that links up all the pencil marks and thus create a profile of aspects of how you perceive the AIDS patient. This will allow you to notice similarities and differences when you compare your ratings with those of your colleagues. The ticks on each dimension may also be given a numerical value which would further aid analysis of data. Statistical analysis could be used to process the data and establish statistical differences between individuals and groups of subjects.

Evaluation: Discuss and compare your findings with those of your colleagues. How could you analyse data collected from a group of people? Is this a method that you could use in your own research project?

As another level of evaluation, it is useful, before you finish the activity, to note down:

(a) what you learned from doing the activity,
(b) how you will use what you learned,
(c) how what you have learned relates to what you have read, and
(d) what you need to learn next.

Delphi Method

The Delphi Method is used to quantify the judgements of experts, to assess priorities, or to produce long-range forecasts. Linstone and Turoff (1975) suggest, amongst other things, that the Delphi Method is useful as a means of:

- Gathering current and historical data not accurately known or available:
- Examining the significance of historical events;
- Evaluating possible budget options;
- Exploring planning options;
- planning curriculum developments;
- looking at the pros and cons of policy options.

The Delphi Method, in essence, involves the asking of a group of experts in a particular field to offer information about a particular topic. Out of the material that is generated, a questionnaire is developed, which is then sent out to that same panel of experts. This cyclical process is continued until the researcher feels confident that she is obtaining a reasonably comprehensive view of the field. The aim is to produce an outcome that is acceptable to the panel of experts.

Further Reading

Bond, S. and Bond, J. (1982) 'A Delphi survey of clinical nursing research priorities', *Journal of Advanced Nursing*, **7** (6) 565–75.
Davis, B.D. and Burnard, P. (1992) 'Academic levels in nursing', *Journal of Advanced Nursing*, **17**, 1395–400.
Fielding, G. (1984) 'Professional problems of caring for the cancer patient', *International Review of Applied Psychology*, **33**, 545–63.
Goodman, C.M. (1987) 'The Delphi technique: a critique', *Journal of Advanced Nursing*, **12** (6) 729–34.

Case Study Technique

A typical definition of the case study approach is that it is the study of an individual person, usually in a problematic situation and often over a relatively short period of time. In other words, it is a word-picture of one part of a person's life. Examples of the case study would be a portrait of a person's care and experience during their treatment for cancer, or a description of a manager's experience of being displaced during a reorganisation of the management structure.

Case studies offer a 'one off' approach to data collection. They offer a rich source of qualitative and descriptive data which can later be content analysed or stand on their own as examples of a particular life-situation.

Many nurses are familiar with being asked to prepare a case study. Normally, in the context of research, a case study would be a study of greater depth than would normally be true of nurse's case studies. Considerably more detail would be collected in a research project and the analysis of the data would be more stringent.

Further Reading

Bromley, D.B. (1986) *The Case-Study Method in Psychology and Related Disciplines*, Wiley, Chichester.
Yin, R.K. (1989) *Case Study Research: Design and Methods*, 2nd edn, Sage, London.

Use of Diaries and Journals

Diaries and journals are descriptions of activities, experiences and feelings, written during a particular time-span. For example, a group of ward sisters may be asked to keep a diary and record their work activities for a period of two months. The information gained in this way can be a rich source of descriptive data. This method is an example of self-reporting.

Further Reading

Henerson, M.E., Morris, L.L. and Fitz-Gibbon, C.T. (1987) *How to Measure Attitudes*, Sage, Beverly Hills, California.
Ruffing-Rahal, M.A. (1986) 'Personal documents and personal theory development', *Advances in Nursing Science*, **8** (3) 50–70.
Woods, N.F. (1981) 'The health diary as an instrument for nursing research: problems and promise', *Western Journal of Nursing Research*, **3** (1) 76–92.

CONCLUSION

These are some other methods of data collection. They have not necessarily been used as frequently in nursing research as those described in the previous chapter but all offer interesting and valuable methods of collecting data. In the final information box, in this chapter, we draw your attention to yet more methods that can be used. The overriding principle in selecting a method is that it should be the one that most clearly offers you the data that can answer your research question or help to solve your research problem. It is wise to become familiar with a wide range of such methods and to note how other researchers, before you, have chosen their methods. In this way you will gradually become more critical of other people's work: a vital aspect of the research process.

Learning Check

If You are Working on Your Own

Read through the notes that you have kept whilst completing the exercises in this chapter and consider the following questions:

- What new knowledge have I gained?
- What new skills have I developed?
- How has my thinking about research changed?
- What do I need to do now?

Check that you have made reference cards for any new references that you have found whilst working on the exercises in this chapter.

If You are Working in a Small Group

Pair off and nominate one of you as A and one of you as B. For five minutes, A talks to B about what she has learned and A listens. This should *not* be a conversation: B's only role is to listen. After five minutes, roles are reversed and B talks to A about what she has learned and A listens. After the second five minutes, re-form into a group and discuss the experience.

If You are a Tutor and/or Facilitator

- Use the above pairs exercise with the group you are working with.
- Hold two 'rounds' in which each person in turn says *(a)* what she liked least about doing the activities and *(b)* what she liked most about doing the activities.

8

Methods of Analysing Data

Aims of this Chapter

These are to:

- Examine methods of analysing data quantitatively;
- Examine methods of analysing data qualitatively;
- To explore combinations of the two approaches;
- To aid the selection of an appropriate method of data analysis for your project.

Introduction

In the two previous chapters, we considered the various methods of collecting data that are available to the researcher. We noted, also, that very often the data collection method is intimately tied to the method of analysis – so much so that on occasions it was difficult, in those chapters, to separate the two. This raises the very important issue that has been alluded to before: methods of analysis must always be considered alongside methods of data collection.

In this chapter we consider two broad approaches to data analysis:

- quantitative and
- qualitative.

Before you work through this chapter, it may be helpful to re-read the sections on the differences between quantitative and qualitative approaches to research, outlined in Chapter 4. It will be recalled that an important difference, in terms of outcome, was that *quantitative* research tends to generate data in the form of numbers. *Qualitative* research tends to generate data that is made up of blocks of text that are interpreted in various ways. The purpose of the analysis, in both cases, however, is to identify patterns or trends emerging from the data. In addition, the researcher must carry out various checks to ensure that these patterns or trends are both *reliable* and *valid* findings (see Chapter 6). In this chapter, the two types of data analysis, quantitative and qualitative are discussed separately. In the conclusion to this chapter, we explore, briefly, the notion of combining the two approaches.

8.1 Quantitative Analysis

What You Need to Read

This should include the following:

Goulding, S. (1987) 'Analysis and Presentation of Information', in Bell, J., *Doing Your Research Project: A Guide for First-Time Researchers in Education and Social Science*, Open University Press, Milton Keynes, pp. 103–23.

Reid, N.G. and Boore, J.R.P. (1987) *Research Methods and Statistics in Health Care*, Arnold, London.

Waltz, C.F., Strickland, O.L. and Lenz, E.R. (1984) *Measurement in Nursing Research*, F.A. Davis, Philadelphia.

Types of Quantitative Analysis

By the end of this section you will have discovered:

- Some common terms used in quantitative analysis;
- Some of the common test used in quantitative analysis;
- Whether or not any of these methods are useful to you in analysing your data.

Exercise 8.1

Aim of the exercise: To explore common terms used in quantitative analysis.

Planning stage: You can do this exercise with a small group of colleagues, friends or students. Allow yourself plenty of time to complete the exercise and make notes of what you do, as you go. If you work with friends of colleagues, decide whether you will all carry out similar tasks or you will divide up the work between you.

Equipment/resources required: Notebook, pen and access to a nursing library.

What to do: Work in small groups of two or three. Divide up the terms listed below, so that each sub-group has two or three terms to consider. Go to the library and select a range of books on research methods. Then consider the terms and write short notes on what they mean. The books recommended above will help you to make a start on this task.

- Statistics: descriptive and inferential
- Nominal scales
- Ordinal scales
- Interval scales
- Ratio scales
- Variable
- Discrete and continuous variable
- Mean
- Mode
- Standard deviation
- Normal distribution
- Parametric and non-parametric tests
- Median
- Cumulative frequency.

Note down other words that are unfamiliar to you and note down their meaning.
Return to the larger group and discuss your findings.
Now break into small groups again and find examples from the literature of the following ways of presenting numerical data:

- Graph
- Pie charts
- Tables
- Histograms
- Bar charts
- Percentage component bar chart.

Return to the larger group and pin up photocopies of the examples that you found. Discuss the ways in which these methods of presentation have been used and why one method is sometimes more appropriately used than another.

Evaluation: Discuss your findings and your progress with your colleagues and a tutor. What sort of data do you think your research project will generate? Consider to what degree quantitative methods of analysis will be appropriate for your project. Consider some of the advantages and disadvantages of the quantitative approach and link your discussion of these issues with the earlier chapter in this book which compares and contrasts the two approaches to research.

As another level of evaluation, it is useful, before you finish the activity, to note down:

(a) what you learned from doing the activity
(b) how you will use what your learned,
(c) how what you have learned relates to what you have read, and
(d) what you need to learn next.

Quantitative Analysis

Quantitative analysis is nearly always analysis of figures. Usually the easiest way of working with lots of figures is by putting them into 'rows and columns'. For this reason, a computer is often the best way of working with numerical data. At least two possibilities open up here. First, numerical data can be stored and, to some extent, manipulated with a *spreadsheet* program. Examples of these include Excel, Quattro Pro for Windows and PlanPerfect. A spreadsheet program allows you to enter numbers into series of rows and columns and then to perform simple and complex calculations on those rows and columns. The findings from those calculations can be converted into a variety of tables and charts or even transferred into a word processing program for further work.

The alternative to working with a spreadsheet is to put your numerical data into a statistical program. This works in a similar way to a spreadsheet application but it also allows for the use of far more complex statistical calculations. Examples of such packages are SPSS for Windows, C-Stat, Unistat and Systat for Windows. Again, all of these programs allow you to produce charts and tables from your findings. An important point is that you should always know *why* you are using a particular statistical test before you ask the program to run it. Computer programs will run statistical tests on any lists of figures but the results of indiscrimate computing can lead to findings that are nonsensical.

Alternatively, if you do not have access to or do not use a computer, you can work with quantitative data on sheets of paper and with a calculator. Again, the idea of rows and columns is a useful one and most modern calculators will allow you to do a range of statistical tests.

The principles of quantitative analysis can be simplified as follows:

1st stage: Findings are grouped together in rows and columns. This is sometimes referred to as the presentation of 'raw' data.

2nd stage: The researcher looks for consistent trends and patterns in the data and sees how the findings are distributed throughout the sample. Descriptive statistics can be used here in the form of frequency counts, means, modes and standard deviations.

3rd stage: The research looks for *particular* trends and patterns. For example, he or she may look at differences between sexes or age groups. The researcher may use a range of statistical tests to verify his or her findings.

4th stage: The researcher presents the findings in a series of charts or tables.

5th stage: The researcher offers *interpretations* or *explanations* of the findings and writes the final research report to communicate his or her findings with others.

These are only *general* guidelines. You need to read more widely on all the possible stages that a quantitative researcher may use in analysing his or her data.

Example

The following short questionnaire is given to 20 people. Each respondent fills in his or her questionnaire and each question on the questionnaire has five possible answers. The first possible answer (strongly agree) is assigned a 1, the second possible answer (agree) is assigned a 2, the third possible answer (uncertain) is assigned a 3 and so on. The example, below, shows how one respondent filled in the questionnaire.

1. Primary nursing is a useful way of organising nursing work.

Strongly Agree	Agree	Uncertain	Disagree	Strongly Disagree	LEAVE BLANK
1 ✓	2	3	4	5	

2. All nurses should use a nursing model to plan their nursing care.

Strongly Agree	Agree	Uncertain	Disagree	Strongly Disagree	LEAVE BLANK
1 ✓	2	3	4	5	

3. Student nurses generally receive excellent training in the use of nursing models.

Strongly Agree	Agree	Uncertain	Disagree	Strongly Disagree	LEAVE BLANK
1	2 ✓	3	4	5	

4. Nursing models are unnecessarily complicated.

Strongly Agree	Agree	Uncertain	Disagree	Strongly Disagree	LEAVE BLANK
1 ✓	2	3	4	5	

5. Primary nursing is not an appropriate approach to nursing in the community.

Strongly Agree	Agree	Uncertain	Disagree	Strongly Disagree	LEAVE BLANK
1	2	3	4 ✓	5	

After all the questionnaires have been filled in, the researcher 'scores' them by inserting the number of the ticked box in the 'leave blank' box. This facility is particularly useful if large numbers of questionnaires are being handled.

Once all the questionnaire items have been scored in this way, the researcher transfers all the scores to the main score sheet. This makes use of the 'rows and columns' arrangement referred to above. The numbered grid allows all of the answers to each question in all of the questionnaires to be grouped together in a single sheet. Alternatively, these numbers could be typed into a spreadsheet or statistics program on a computer. Any 'missing' scores (where the respondent has missed answering a particular item) is allocated the number 9 to distinguish it from any 'actual' answers.

	Quest 1	Quest 2	Quest 3	Quest 4	Quest 5
Respondent 1	1	1	2	1	4
Respondent 2	2	1	4	3	3
Respondent 3	2	2	4	3	3
Respondent 4	1	2	5	4	3
Respondent 5	3	2	5	2	3
Respondent 6	1	2	5	1	1
Respondent 7	3	3	5	3	9
Respondent 8	1	2	4	1	2
Respondent 9	2	4	2	1	2
Respondent 10	1	1	5	1	1
Respondent 11	2	3	3	3	4
Respondent 12	1	5	5	1	5
Respondent 13	1	3	9	1	5

	Quest 1	Quest 2	Quest 3	Quest 4	Quest 5
Respondent 14	1	3	5	3	2
Respondent 15	4	3	4	3	3
Respondent 16	4	2	4	2	4
Respondent 17	2	4	5	4	1
Respondent 18	3	9	9	3	4
Respondent 19	1	2	3	1	1
Respondent 20	2	1	4	1	1

After this, the researcher can determine, either by hand or through the use of a computer, a 'frequency count'. This means that he or she works out how many '5's there were as a response to question 1 (and, therefore, how many people answered 'strongly agree' to it), how many '4's and so on. From this type of frequency count, if he had a large number of responses, he could work out the *percentage* of respondents' responses to all of the questionnaire items. After this, he could illustrate those percentages in a *bar chart*. Figure 8.1 shows a frequency count for question 1, from the above grid.

It is important to note that none of the columns in the grid can be added up: the figures in the boxes are used merely as 'markers' to act as a shorthand for answers to questions. It would have been almost as easy to allocate *letters* to each of the possible answers to the questions and then it would have been very apparent that the columns could not be added up! On the other hand, it is easy to see how all the 5's, all the 4's, 3's, 2's and 1's in each column could be calculated and how '9's would have to be discounted. It may also be easy to see how items of data soon mount up. This was a very short questionnaire given to a small number of respondents and yet it yielded 100 separate items of data. Larger questionnaires and larger samples of respondents are nearly always more easily handled with a computer program.

Question 1: *Primary nursing is a useful way of organising nursing work.*	Numbers of responses
Strongly agree (1's)	9
Agree (2's)	6
Uncertain (3's)	3
Disagree (4's)	2
Strongly disagree (5's)	0
Total number of responses	20

Figure 8.1

Further Reading

Burnard, P. (1993) *Personal Computing for Health Professionals*, Chapman & Hall, London.

Polger, S. and Thomas, S.A. (1991) *Introduction to Research in the Health Sciences*, 2nd edn, Churchill Livingstone, Melbourne.

Reid, N.G. and Boore, J.R.P. (1987) *Research Methods and Statistics in Health Care*, Edward Arnold, Sevenoaks.

Rose, D. and Sullivan, O. (1993) *Introducing Data Analysis for Social Scientists*, Open University Press, Milton Keynes.

Rowntree, D. (1981) *Statistics without Tears: A Primer for Non-Mathematicians*, Penguin, Harmondsworth.

Exercise 8.2

Aim of the exercise: To explore some simple statistical calculations.

Planning stage: This activity is best carried out by the individual working on her own. Allow yourself plenty of time to complete the exercise and make notes of what you do, as you go.

122

Equipment/resources required: Notebook, pen and access to a nursing library, calculator.

What to do: Consider the following table:

Monthly discharge rate from an acute admission psychiatric ward over a two year period.

					Months of the year							
	J	F	M	A	M	J	J	A	S	O	N	D
Year 1	27	24	30	30	21	24	29	28	20	25	24	22
Year 2	29	30	26	24	20	29	30	24	22	23	23	20

Now calculate the following:

• The mean discharge rate over the two-year period.
• The mean discharge rate for year one and for year two.
• The mean discharge rate for each month of the year, over the two-year period.

Now draw a bar chart that illustrates the mean discharge rate for each month of the year, over the two-year period.

Now calculate the following:

• The frequency of each of the values,

Convert these into a pie chart.

Now calculate:

• The median for this set of values;
• The cumulative frequency for this set of values.

If you experience any problems with these calculations, refer to: Reid, N.G. and Boore, J.R.P. (1987) *Research Methods and Statistics in Health Care*, Arnold, London.

Evaluation: Check through your answers with a group of colleagues and with a tutor.

As another level of evaluation, it is useful, before you finish the activity, to note down:

(a) what you learned from doing the activity
(b) how you will use what you learned,
(c) how what you have learned relates to what you have read, and
(d) what you need to learn next.

Exercise 8.3

Aim of the exercise: To explore problems associated with the use of statistical arguments.

Planning stage: You can do this exercise with a small group of colleagues, friends or students. Allow yourself plenty of time to complete the exercise and make notes of what you do, as you go. If you work with friends or colleagues, decide whether you will all carry out similar tasks or you will divide up the work between you.

Equipment / resources required: Notebook, pen and access to a nursing library.

What to do: Read the following proposition and the rationale that accompanies it. The rationale offers an explanation of a statistical table and the proposition is based on how a statistician can interpret a set of statistics. Read the passage through and then decide for yourself if the proposition is a valid one. If you come to the conclusion that it is, think again!

This is an exercise in the art of reading statistics. The discussion focuses on one proposition and is divided into two parts. The first offers a statistical argument in support of the proposition. The second offers a critique of that statistical argument. The critique is developed by noting any assumptions, inconsistencies or fallacies in the statistical argument and building the discussion around them.

The art of reading statistics is to place them in an appropriate context and then to interpret them by reference to that background. This requires considerable knowledge of the relevant subject areas, so read the discussions critically and carefully!

The Proposition: Marriage is fatal for the man.

The Supporting Argument: It is no longer socially unacceptable for a couple to enter into an unhallowed and extra-legal partnership in which they live together as man and wife. This change in attitude developed from the appreciation by a substantial proportion of adults of the real consequences of marriage. It is, quite simply, that marriage is fatal for the man. The table below demonstrates this fact conclusively.

Women outnumber men. However, they do not do so over all age groups. In the younger age group men outnumber women. As men grow older this situation is reversed by their death rate increasing more rapidly than the death rate for women. The change occurs when men and women are in the fifth decade of their lives. Its effect is that a 3 per cent surplus of men in the younger age group is converted to a 23 per cent surplus of women in the older age groups.

A single factor produces the change. A common experience of the factor kills men more quickly than women. That factor is marriage. Is it sufficiently widespread to produce the change? And, by the time the change occurs men have experienced marriage for a sufficient length of time for it to produce the change. The extent of the change is accounted for by the virulence of marriage.

Population of England and Wales, mid-1971 ('000s)

Age	Male	Female	Total
0–4	2 009	1 911	3 920
5–14	3 980	3 776	7 756
15–19	1 715	1 640	3 355
20–29	3 526	3 469	6 995
30–44	4 340	4 258	8 598
45–74	7 437	8 506	15 943
75 and over	713	1 534	2 247
Totals	23 720	25 094	48 814

Source: The Registrar General's Statistical Review of England and Wales, 1971, part 2, 1973, Table A6: 10–11.

Evaluation: Now evaluate the above argument, either as individuals working alone or with colleagues of friends in a group setting. Can you spot any problems in the above set of arguments? Do not give up too quickly. The development of critical skills is an important one. If you cannot puzzle out the problems, read the paragraphs below. If you do identify problems, read the paragraphs to confirm your own arguments or to develop other perspectives on the problem.

A Critique of the Supporting Argument

The statistical argument implies that the table shows what happened over time. But the table shows the situation at a single point in time, namely, mid-1971. It therefore does not show that 'as men grow older . . . a 3 per cent surplus of men in the younger age groups is converted into a 23 per cent surplus of women in the older age groups'. The only statistics which can show whether such a conversion occurs are those which compare the same group of men and women over all age groups. They are obtained by following the group throughout its life.

As an illustration of what such statistics would show, consider the '75 and over' age group. It contains the largest surplus of women. Notice that a man aged 75 years in 1971 would have been 20 years old in 1916, that is, about the middle of the First World War. Clearly, the surplus of women is explained, in part at least, by the ravages on the battlefields of that war.

Now consider the second oldest age group. It is the only other age group in which women outnumber men. Notice that a man aged 50 years in 1971 would have been 20 years old in 1942: this is near the middle of the Second World War. Once again, the surplus of women is explained, in part at least, by battlefield deaths.

In both age groups the differences are further reduced by the residual effects of the two wars. These effects include the premature deaths of men who survived the wards as battlefield casualties and as prisoners of war. They also include the premature deaths of men who were not conscripted because of ill health.

The statistical argument states that 'a common experience . . . kills men more quickly than women'. This implies that a causal relationship exists when two factors are each experienced by a large proportion of the individuals in a group. In other words, it implies that a strong statistical relationship denotes a causal relationship. In fact, a strong statistical relationship does nothing of the kind. All any statistical relationship can ever do is show the observed strength of a causal relationship established by theory. The reason is quite simple. Statistical relationships are easy to manufacture.

As an example, suppose that in a group of 10 women, 8 are married and 8 wear jeans. At least 6, i.e. at least 75 per cent of the married women wear jeans. Consequently there is a strong statistical relationship between being married and wearing jeans. As this is a fabricated relationship, it is quite meaningless, despite its apparent strength. If this were not so, the relationship would show that only married women normally wear jeans. In this case the converse would also be true. This is that single women do not normally wear jeans. We know that neither is true.

Clearly, the statistical argument is defective on two major counts. It is also defective on a third count. The data are inappropriate. The comparison should be of married men and women, not all men and women. And, the measure of the effect of marriage should be the length of marriage at death, not the age of the individual.

Individually the deficiencies raise doubts about the validity of the statistical argument. Together they establish that it is totally unsound. The statistical argument therefore does not support the proposition. It does not establish that marriage is fatal for the man, even though this may well be the case.

As another level of evaluation, it is useful, before you finish the activity, to note down:

(a) what you learned from doing the activity
(b) how you will use what you learned,
(c) how what you have learned relates to what you have read, and
(d) what you need to learn next.

8.2   Qualitative Analysis

What You Need to Read

This should include the following:

Burgess, R.G. (1984) *In the Field: An Introduction to Field Research*, Allen & Unwin, London.
Lofland, J. and Lofland, L. (1984) *Analysing Social Settings*, 2nd edn, Wadsworth, Belmont, California.
Taylor, S.J. and Bogdan, R. (1984) *Introduction to Qualitative Research Methods: The Search for Meanings*, 2nd edn, Wiley, New York.

Exploring Qualitative Analysis

By the end of this section you will have discovered:

- How to identify different frameworks for analysing qualitative data;
- Whether or not any of these methods are useful to you in analysing your data.

Qualitative Analysis

The qualitative researcher starts with a different *sort* of data to the quantitative researcher in that he or she is nearly always working with *text*. Also, he or she may or may not start with a different set of assumptions about the purpose and nature of the research process. The philosophical positions of the two sorts of researchers may or may not be quite different.

In the end, all qualitative researchers have to make sense of what can be large amounts of text – often in the form of transcripts. Like all researchers, he or she is searching for patterns and groupings in those data, in an attempt to understand what other people think, feel and experience. The problem for the qualitative researcher is staying 'true' to the respondent. Whilst the quantitative researcher is dealing with numbers, the qualitative researcher is also dealing with the difficult area of personal meanings. Just as there are computer programs to help in quantitative analysis, so there are others (such as The Ethnograph) that help the researcher to organise and analyse qualitative data. The following stages represent some of the stages that may be worked through by a qualitative researcher:

Stage 1: The data is gathered into a manageable format – usually a series of transcriptions.

Stage 2: A decision is made about a structured method of handling and analysing the data (e.g. ground theory or phenomenological analysis).

Stage 3: The data is analysed into smaller chunks, meaning units or categories.

Stage 4: The researcher looks for common themes and patterns.

Stage 5: The researcher checks the validity of his or her analysis both with other researchers, with the informants and with the available literature.

Stage 6: The researcher offer accounts and explanations of *why* the data group together in this way.

Stage 7: If required, the researcher refines old theories in the light of the findings or develops new theories.

Stage 8: The researcher writes up and communicate his or her findings.

These are only *general* guidelines. You need to read more widely on all the possible stages that a qualitative researcher may use in analysing his or her data.

Example

Ten semi-structured interviews were conducted with nursing lecturers and extracts from two interviews are illustrated below. The interviews were about assessing teaching in a college of nursing.

Extract One

RESEARCHER: *... and what sorts of methods of assessment do you use, yourself?*
INTERVIEWEE: *I ask the students, I suppose. I ask them at the end of the block of study how they felt about the teaching. I mean, I suppose its not very scientific ... sometimes I give them a questionnaire to fill in. It's not easy. The books suggest that you should regularly assess your teaching so that you can improve learning but I am not sure that the connection between teaching and learning has been established. Not completely.*

Extract Two

RESEARCHER: *... how do you* know *that the students like your teaching?*
INTERVIEWEE: *They tell me! They tell me that the like the way I do things. That's the most important thing, really – that the students feel OK about what happens. Some of my colleagues use more formal approaches but I'm not sure that they get anything more out of it. One interviews each of the students at the end of the block – a sort of tutorial. I think they tell him what he wants to hear ...*

Following the interviews, the researcher read through each of the transcripts and identified a range of categories that appeared to account for *everything* that each interviewee talked about. The complete range of categories was as follows (bear in mind that the two examples, above, are only *small extracts* from *two* of the interviews):

Student's views of teaching
Lecturer's views of teaching
The 'feel-good' factor
Assessment procedures
Student assessment
Personal preferences
Theories about assessment.

After these categories had been developed, the researcher returned to each of his interview transcripts and divided them up according to those categories. The section, below, shows how some parts of the extracts, above, fitted into the category system that had been developed. In 'real life', the process of selecting categories and making sure they are exhaustive of everything that has been discussed in interviews is a laborious and complicated one and one that needs considerable time and concentration. Also, the category system needs to be checked with other colleagues and with the interviewees for face validity. It is important that the category system that you have developed is a valid one and that there is clear evidence that you did not simply 'dream up' the categories.

Category: The 'feel-good' factor
'That's the most important thing, really – that the students feel OK about what happens.'

Category: Theories about assessment
'The books suggest that you should regularly assess your teaching so that you can improve learning but I am not sure that the connection between teaching and learning has been established. Not completely.'

Category: Assessment procedures
'I ask the students, I suppose. I ask them at the end of the block of study how they felt about the teaching. I mean, I suppose its not very scientific . . .'

' . . . sometimes I give them a questionnaire to fill in. It's not easy.'

'They tell me! They tell me that the like the way I do things.'

This example is *one* example of a form of *content analysis* of interviews. As we have discussed at other points in this chapter, there are many *other* ways of analysing qualitative data.

Further Reading

Charmaz, K. (1990) 'Discovering chronic illness: using grounded theory', *Social Science and Medicine*, **30** (11) 1161–72.

Gilbert, N. (1993) *Researching Social Life*, Sage, London.

Patten, M.Q. (1990) *Qualitative Evaluation and Research Methods*, Sage, London.

Tesch, R. (1990) *Qualitative Research: Analysis Types and Software Tools*, Falmer, London.

Spinelli, E. (1989) *The Interpreted World: An Introduction to Phenomenological Psychology*, Sage, London.

Wertz, F. (1983) 'Some constituents of descriptive psychological reflection', *Human Studies*, **6** 35–51.

Learning More About Quantitative and Qualitative Research

These are some routes to learning more about the subject:

• Evening classes at colleges and extra-mural departments of universities;
• Asking for a course of lectures on the topic in the school or college of nursing;
• Using learning packages;
• Working with a research supervisor;
• Reading;
• Open University programmes on the television;
• Lecturers and seminar groups;
• Working alongside an experienced researcher;
• Taking part in collecting data for a researcher;
• Volunteering as a respondent in a research project;
• Learning computer programs to analyse data – both qualitative and quantitative.

Exercise 8.4

Aim of the exercise: To explore qualitative analysis of data.

Planning stage: You can do this exercise on your own or in the company of a small group of colleagues, friends or students. Allow yourself plenty of time to complete the exercise and make notes of what you do, as you go. If you work with friends or colleagues, decide whether or not you will all carry out similar tasks or you will divide up the work between you.

Equipment / resources required: Notebook, pen and access to a nursing library.

What to do: Read through the following extract from an interview with a patient. The interview comes from a study of patient's perceptions of the information they have been given about their illness. As you read through, consider what *sorts* of statements the person is making and whether or not a number of the statements fall into certain groups of themes. For example, does the person refer to certain grades of staff, does she talk about how she feels and so on?

> *I've been on the ward about six weeks now . . . no one really tells you very much . . . I mean, the doctor talked to my husband and my daughter. He didn't talk to me. I get very depressed about it all. Sometimes I don't sleep all that well. Mind you, I don't sleep very well at home, either. The sister's very good. She always answers any questions I have but she doesn't seem to want to talk to me about what's wrong with me. . . . I think I know though. My daughter always tells me not to worry. I get scared, sometimes. Why won't they tell me?*
>
> *I go to physiotherapy twice a week. Susan, down there, always says how well I'm doing. I don't think she really knows the whole story. She's more interested in my leg! I like it down there, though . . . I meet a lot of other people. You can talk to other people because they're in the same boat. I don't get so fed up down there. It's the company, I think. Mind you, my husband tries to talk to me. It's not the same in hospital, though.*

The aim of a qualitative analysis of this sort of data is to classify as many statements of units of meaning from the data so that the researcher can make sense of it. The generation of categories of response also allows for comparisons to be made between different sets of data.

Read through the passage above, again, and try to organise phrases from the passage under the following headings that have been generated from the data:

- Types of people discussed
- Feelings expressed
- Activities
- Levels of communication
- Comments about being in hospital
- Comparisons of hospital life with other aspects of life
- Theories about communication in hospital.
- Comments about illness.

Example

- Feelings expressed:
  'I get very depressed about it all'
  'I get scared, sometimes'
  'I don't get so fed up down there' (physiotherapy)

This is one stage, in one approach to qualitative analysis.

Now read the following material on qualitative analysis and compare the method you have just explored with other qualitative methods. Also note how the method described here fits into the overall research plan. For example, what could you do after you have discovered categories in the data? How would you write up your analysis?
    The reading material is:

Melia, K.M. (1987) *Learning and Working: The Occupational Socialisation of Nurses*, Tavistock, London.
Hycner, R.H. (1985) 'Some guidelines for the phenomenological analysis of interview data', *Human Studies*, **8**, 279–303.
Watson, J. (1985) *Nursing: Human Science and Human Care: A Theory of Nursing*: Appleton-Century-Crofts, Connecticut.

Evaluation: Discuss your category system with your colleagues. Consider whether or not a method such as this would be an appropriate way to analyse the data that will emerge out of your research project.
    As another level of evaluation, it is useful, before you finish the activity, to note down:

(a) what you learned from doing the activity,
(b) how you will use what you learned,
(c) how what you have learned relates to what you have read, and
(d) what you need to learn next.

CONCLUSION

You have now explored two approaches to handling data. From a philosophical point of view, the quantitative and qualitative approaches start from very different assumptions about the nature of research. From a practical point of view, however, it is possible to use and combine both approaches.

For instance, it is entirely possible to undertake both a qualitative analysis of an interview, followed by a detailed content analysis. In this way, both approaches are combined.

Learning Check

If You are Working on Your Own

Read through the notes that you have kept whilst completing the exercises in this chapter and consider the following questions:

- What new knowledge have I gained?
- What new skills have I developed?
- How has my thinking about research changed?
- What do I need to do now?

Check that you have made reference cards for any new references that you have found whilst working on the exercises in this chapter.

If You are Working in a Small Group

Pair off and nominate one of you as A and one of you as B. For five minutes, A talks to B about what she has learned and A listens. This should *not* be a conversation: B's only role is to listen. After five minutes, roles are reversed and B talks to A about what she has learned and A listens. After the second five minutes, re-form into a group a discuss the experience.

If You are a Tutor and/or Facilitator

- Use the above pairs exercise with the group you are working with.
- Hold two 'rounds' in which each person in turn says *(a)* what she liked least about doing the activities and *(b)* what she liked most about doing the activities.

9

Undertaking the Research Project

Aims of this Chapter

These are:

- To enable you to structure your time;
- To consider aspects of supervision;
- To plan and work consistently through your project.

Introduction

All the previous chapters have focused on discrete parts of the research process. Our aim in this chapter is to pull the threads together to enable you to work through the project as a whole.

What You Need to Read

This should include the following:

Armitage, S. and Rees, C. (1988) 'Student projects: a practical framework', *Nurse Education Today*, **8**, 289–95.
British Psychological Society (1987) 'Code of practice on supervision, preparation and examination of doctoral theses in departments of psychology,' *Bulletin of the British Psychological Society*, **40**, 250–4.
Hawthorne, P.J. (1981) 'Supervision of dissertations of undergraduate nursing students', *Nursing Times*, **77** (8) 29–30: Occasional Paper.
Howard, K. and Sharp, J.A. (1983) *The Management of a Student Research Project*, Gower, Aldershot.

Madder, R. (1988) 'Encouraging students to be research minded', *Nurse Education Today*, **8**, 30–5.

9.1 Time Management

By the end of this section you will have discovered:

- How to plan your work;
- How to use time effectively.

Exercise 9.1

Aim of the exercise: Planning your research project in terms of time.

Planning stage: This exercise should be carried out in a small group. Allow yourself plenty of time to complete the exercise and make notes of what you do, as you go. If you work with friends or colleagues, decide whether you will all carry out similar tasks or you will divide up the work between you.

Equipment / resources required: Notebook, pen and access to a nursing library.

What to do: You are going to use the process know as 'outlining'. First, jot down on a sheet of paper, the broad stages of your research project, e.g.:

- planning stage
- searching the literature
- collecting data
- analysing data
- writing up.

Now consider how much time you think you will have available for each broad state and write that time-allowance down next to each heading.
    Then take each of these stages in turn and write down sub-tasks that have to be completed in order to complete that stage and time that sub-task, e.g.:

- Planning stage (two weeks)
- Identifying area of interest (two days)
- Choosing research question/problem (two days)
- Discussion and contract-setting with supervisor (two days)
- Identifying resources and constraints (two days)
- Drawing up timetable for the whole of the project (two days)
- Negotiating access to data collection site (two days).

Notice how quickly your time gets used up! When you have completed each stage, identify to what degree you need to cut back on certain sub-stages. It is useful if you consider your planning under the following three headings:

- What *must* be done
- What *should* be done
- What *could* be done (if time is available)

After you have completed this planning task, draw up a 'master plan' of your research project, showing how aspects of your work will fit into a time scale (see Figure 9.1). Notice that some tasks will run concurrently with others or overlap with others.

WEEK ONE	WEEK TWO
Mon Tues Wed Thurs Frid Sat Sun	Mon Tues Wed Thurs Frid Sat Sun

Figure 9.1   Example of a master plan for a two-week research project

Evaluation: Discuss your plan with your supervisor and with your colleagues. Ask them to play 'devil's advocate' and look for problems in your planning. Time spent at this stage is time well spent in that an organised approach will help your project to run smoothly.

As another level of evaluation, it is useful, before you finish the activity, to note down:

(a) what you learned from doing the activity,
(b) how you will use what you learned,
(c) how what you have learned relates to what you have read, and
(d) what you need to learn next.

Aspects of Time Management

DO:

- Keep detailed notes as you progress through your project.
- Be disciplined in your approach: if you plan to do something, DO IT!
- Keep your reference cards up-to-date and make sure that ALL details of the reference are recorded.
- Be systematic in your work.
- Try not to attempt the same task twice. If you have planned adequately, you should be able to complete a task in one go.
- Keep in touch with your supervisor.

DON'T

- Don't leave everything to the last minute: work through your project systematically,
- Don't expect your supervisor to do your project for you!
- Don't expect your supervisor to see you without an appointment: she has a busy schedule as well.
- Don't expect your local library to have all the references you require; plan ahead for books and articles that may take some time to get.

In summarising issues relating to time management, Godefroy and Clark (1989) make the following points:

- Programme no more than 10 items per day
- Divide complex and demanding tasks into more easily programmable sub-activities.
- Learn to make an accurate estimate of the time needed for each task.

- Be ambitious but don't overload yourself.
- Programme only 60 per cent of your time.
- Revise your plan regularly.
- Finish each task before going onto the next.

Robson (1993) makes the following points about time management and doing your research project:

> Any real world study must obviously take serious note of real world constraints. Your choice of research focus must be realistic in terms of the time and resources that you have available. If you have a maximum of three weeks you can devote to the project, you choose something where you have a good chance of 'getting it out' in that time. Access and cooperation are similarly important, as well as having a good nose for situations where any enquiry is likely to be counter-productive (getting into a sensitive situation involving, say, the siting of a hostel for mentally handicapped adults when your prime aim is to develop community provision is not very sensible if a likely outcome is the stirring up of a hornet's nest).

Budgeting a Research Project

Most diploma and undergraduate research projects will not require special funding. It is expected that you will work out your proposal so that no 'extra' costs are involved. For example, it will probably be anticipated that you will pay for your own paper for questionnaires, do you own typing or word processing and pay for any local travelling that you have to do. As you move on, however, and do postgraduate or become involved in funded projects, you will have to work out a *budget* for the project. Bear in mind, though, that *all* research projects involve *some* costs and it is worth knowing about how professional researchers budget their programmes.

Here are some examples of the sorts of items that need to be costed in a larger-scale research project. If you have occasion to apply for grants, scholarships or awards, it is likely that you will be asked to prepare a statement of projected costs. Not all funding bodies will ask for all of the following details but read them through and see which ones might apply to your own work.

Personnel
- Salary of research assistant (full or part-time)
- Salary of clerical assistant (full or part-time)
- Training of interviewers
- Computer software training for personnel

Travelling expenses
- Travel to interview sites
- Local travel to libraries and appointments
- Travel, fees and accommodation at conferences (national and/or international)

Office equipment
- Computing equipment
- Printers (usually a laser printer)
- Computer software
- Office space
- Telephone rental
- Fax and modem equipment
- Photocopying equipment
- Paper and other stationery

Use of facilities
- Use of library (including searching facilities)
- Use of abstracting services
- Postage

Add-on administrative costs
- Many colleges and universities take a percentage of any research monies that are attracted by their staff. This percentage should be accounted for in any initial budgeting.

Further Reading

Arber, S. (1993) 'The research process', in N. Gilbert (ed.) *Researching Social Life*, Sage, London.

Fineman, S. (1981) 'Funding research: practice and politics', in P. Reason and J. Rowan (eds) *Human Inquiry: A Sourcebook of New Paradigm Research*, Wiley, Chichester.

Pariah, K. (1988) 'Funding nursing research', *Senior Nurse*, **8** (9/10) 12–14.

Tierney, A.J. (1989) 'Grantsmanship: resources for nursing research', *Senior Nurse*, **9** (2) 9.

9.2 Supervision of your Research Project

A supervisor is the person who oversees your research project. He or she will usually be a tutor or lecturer in the department in which you are studying. Supervisors will usually have successfully completed research of their own and may be working on current research projects of their own. They are a valuable resource.

By the end of this section you will have discovered:

- What you can expect of your supervisor;
- What your supervisor can expect of you.

Exercise 9.2

Aim of the exercise: To explore the role of the supervisor

Planning stage: This exercise should be carried out on your own and then your findings discussed in a small group. Allow yourself plenty of time to complete the exercise and make notes of what you do, as you go.

Equipment/resources required: Notebook, pen and access to a nursing library.

What to do: Sit down and write out a list entitled 'What I expect from a supervisor'. You may want to consider such issues as:

- 'She will help me to plan my work'
- 'She will discuss aspects of the methodology'
- 'She will offer constructive criticism of my work', etc.

Now ask your supervisor to undertake a similar exercise. Ask her to write down *two* lists: 'What I can offer as a supervisor' and 'What I expect from you'.

Evaluation: When you have carried out these two task, sit and discuss your roles and negotiate a working relationship for the research project.

As another level of evaluation, it is useful, before you finish the activity, to note down:

(a) what you learned from doing the activity,
(b) how you will use what you learned,
(c) how what you have learned relates to what you have read, and
(d) what you need to learn next.

A Checklist for Achieving Good Research Supervision

The successful completion of a research project is probably one of the most difficult facets of any project. Completing such a project is very much a joint venture involving a research student and a supervisor. Listed below are items which can help promote good supervisory practice.

Supervisor

1. What steps are taken to try and make a good match between a supervisor and the student?
2. Does the supervisor allocate adequate time to meet with the student?
3. Does the supervisor insist on regular written material throughout the project?
4. Does the supervisor insist on setting aims for the next meeting?
5. Has the supervisor demonstrated how to make systematic records?
6. Does the supervisor help the student to select problems, stimulate and enthuse the student and provide a steady stream of scientific ideas and guidance?

Student

1. Have you planned your project satisfactorily?
2. Have you identified key problem areas?
3. Do you understand the relevant literature?
4. Do you keep accurate and systematic records of what you read and what you do?
5. Do you write up your project in small increments as you progress from beginning to end?
6. Do you approach your supervisor when requiring help, giving adequate time for an appointment to be made and, where appropriate, specifying the problem?

Several of these items are adapted from the guidelines provided by SERC (1983).

Further Reading

Elton, L. and Pope, M. (1989) 'Research supervision: the value of collegiality', *Cambridge Journal of Education*, **19** (3) 267–76.
Sheehan, J. (1993) 'Issues in the supervision of postgraduate research students in nursing', *Journal of Advanced Nursing*, **18**, 880–5.

Conclusion

In this book we have tried to show you that you can do research. The main theme running through this particular chapter has been the need to be planned and systematic in your approach. Whilst research is not easy, it is easier if you plan it well. Also, the need to be systematic is part of the research process itself: you cannot claim validity for your project if you cannot account for certain aspects of it.

Further, the systematic approach needs to be sustained. As with all things, there are peaks and troughs in any project. The systematic approach will help you to keep going when you are less than enthusiastic about what you are doing. Systematic planning can also point to certain 'maintenance tasks' – filing, checking references and so on – that can help you maintain a sense of impetus.

Note, also, that the efficient planner will think in terms of the 'sub-goals' described above. A sense of achievement will be reinforced by having achieved each of these smaller sub-goals. On the other hand, if you do *not* break down tasks in this way, you may find yourself daunted by the apparent magnitude of the work that is in front of you.

In the final chapter, we consider how to write up your work. If you have planned your project well, this process should be reasonably straightforward: all the hard work will have been done and your systematic notes will allow you to organise your final write-up.

Learning Check

If You are Working on Your Own

Read through the notes that you have kept whilst completing the exercises in this chapter and consider the following questions:

- What new knowledge have I gained?
- What new skills have I developed?
- How has my thinking about research changed?
- What do I need to do now?

Check that you have made reference cards for any new references that you have found whilst working on the exercises in this chapter.

If You are Working in a Small Group

Pair off and nominate one of you as A and one of you as B. For five minutes, A talks to B about what she has learned and A listens. This should *not* be a conversation: B's only role is to listen. After five minutes, roles are reversed and B talks to A about what she has learned and A listens. After the second five minutes, re-form into a group A discuss the experience.

If You are a Tutor and/or Facilitator

- Use the above pairs exercise with the group you are working with.
- Hold two 'rounds' in which each person in turn says *(a)* what she liked least about doing the activities and *(b)* what she liked most about doing the activities.

10

Writing the Research Report

Aims of this Chapter

These are:

- To identify the stages in writing up a research report;
- To consider how to submit a research report to a journal for consideration for publication;
- Feeding back your findings to the participants in your study.

Introduction

All research has to be 'written up'. The reasons for this are fairly clear:

- A research report demonstrates how you have carried out your work and how you reached your conclusions.
- A research report allows you to share your findings with others.
- A research report adds to the body of knowledge in a particular discipline and allows others to criticise your work and to develop it.

You may also want to have your research report considered for publication in a nursing magazine or journal. In this way, your work reaches a wider audience.

What You Need to Read

This should include the following:

Barzun, J. and Graff, H.E. (1977) *The Modern Researcher*, 3rd edn, Harcourt, Brace Jovanovich, New York.
Bell, J. (1987) 'Writing the Report' in Bell, J., *Doing Your Research Project:*

A Guide for First Time Researchers in Education and Social Science, Open University Press, Milton Keynes, pp. 124–35.

Bogdan, R.C. and Biklen, S.K. (1982) *Qualitative Research for Education: An Introduction to Theory and Methods*, Allyn & Bacon, Boston, Massachusetts.

Burnard, P. (1992) *Writing for Health Professionals: A Writer's Manual*, Chapman & Hall, London.

Morris, S. (1988) 'Writing a book: some advice for new authors', *Nurse Education Today*, **8**, 234–8.

10.1 Planning Your Research Report

By the end of this section you will have discovered:

• The structure of a research report;
• How to write clearly;
• How to write for publication.

Exercise 10.1

Aim of the exercise: To explore various ways of structuring a research report

Planning stage: You can do this exercise on your own or in the company of a small group of colleagues, friends or students. Allow yourself plenty of time to complete the exercise and make notes of what you do, as you go. If you work with friends or colleagues, decide whether you will all carry out similar tasks or you will divide up the work between you.

Equipment/resources required: Notebook, pen and access to a nursing library.

What to do: Go to the library and study the following research reports. Make notes under the following headings:

• What headings does the writer use to structure her report?
• What differences are there in writing up a qualitative study and a quantitative study?
• To what degree did illustrations and tables help or hinder your understanding of the research findings?

- What style of write-up would best suit your own work?
- What skills do you need to develop in order to write your own research report?

The studies to review are:

Bogdan, R., Brown, M.A. and Foster, S.B. (1982) 'Be honest but not cruel: staff/parent communication on a neonatal unit', *Human Organisation*, **41** (1) 6–16.

Burnard, P. and Morrison, P. (1988) 'Nurses' perceptions of their interpersonal skills: a descriptive study using six category intervention analysis', *Nurse Education Today*, **8** 266–272.

Melia, K. (1987) *Learning and Working: The Occupational Socialisation of Nurses*, Tavistock, London.

Morrison, P. and le Roux, B. (1987) 'The Practice of Seclusion', *Nursing Times*, **83** (19) 62–6 Occasional Paper.

There is no 'right way' to structure a research report. However, certain headings and sub-headings occur in many studies. If you have followed a logical sequence of events in doing your research, that sequence should guide you to the structuring of your report. Headings that you may want to consider are as follows:

1. Title
2. Summary
3. Precise statement of the scope and aims of the study
4. Rationale for the study
5. Review of the literature
6. Description of methods used
7. Description and presentation of findings
8. Analysis and discussion of findings
9. Conclusions and recommendations
10. References
11. Appendices.

Evaluation: Discuss your findings with your colleagues and decide upon what skills each of you has and what skills each of you needs to acquire in order to write up your study.

   As another level of evaluation, it is useful, before you finish the activity, to note down:

(a) what you learned from doing the activity,
(b) how you will use what you learned,
(c) how what you have learned relates to what you have read, and
(d) what you need to learn next.

10.2 Writing your Report

By the end of this section you will have discovered:

- How to write clearly;
- The materials needed for a write-up;
- How to present your write-up.

Exercise 10.2

Aim of the exercise: To explore approaches to writing a research report.

Planning stage: You can do this exercise on your own or in the company of a small group of colleagues, friends or students. Allow yourself plenty of time to complete the exercise and make notes of what you do, as you go. If you work with friends or colleagues, decide whether you will all carry out similar tasks or you will divide up the work between you.

Equipment/resources required: Notebook, pen and access to a nursing library.

What to do: Go to a college or university library and ask to see copies of student dissertations and/or theses. If you do not have access to such a library, order one or more of the following dissertations/theses from your local library via inter-library loan.

Barker, P. (1988) 'Nursing the patient with major affective disorder', PhD thesis, Dundee College of Technology.
Bauer, I.L. (1993) 'Patients' privacy: an exploratory study of patients' perceptions of their privacy in a German acute care hospital', unpublished PhD thesis, University of Wales College of Medicine.
Burnard, P. (1990) 'Learning from experience: nurse tutors' and student nurses' perceptions of experiential learning', unpublished PhD thesis, University of Wales College of Medicine.
Elkind, A.K. (1980) 'Smoking amongst women with special reference to those training for a profession', PhD thesis, University of Manchester.
Hagan, T. (1988) 'Underutilisation of maternal and child health care', unpublished PhD thesis, Sheffield Hallam University.

McKenna, H. (1992) 'The selection and evaluation of a nursing model for long stay psychiatric patient care', unpublished PhD thesis, University of Ulster.

Morrison, P. (1991) 'The meaning of caring interpersonal relationships in nursing', unpublished PhD thesis, Sheffield Hallam University.

As you look through these dissertations and theses, make notes on the following:

- How are the words laid out on the page: what line-spacing has been used?
- What size margins have been used?
- Are the pages numbered?
- Is there a table of contents?
- Have appendices been used for additional material?
- Is the report written on both sides of the page or only on one?
- Are headings used and, if so, how?
- How is the report bound?
- How is the list of references presented?

Consider, also, whether there are particular rules about the presentation of your research project that are peculiar to your college or school. Sometimes there are written details of how to prepare a research report for your organisation.

Bear in mind that the reports we have asked you to look at are reports submitted for higher degrees. We do not anticipate that you will necessarily be writing in this way. The reports do, however, offer good examples of a standard approach and layout for presenting a written report of a research project.

Evaluation: Discuss with your colleagues your findings and draw up a chart of the necessary considerations that need to be made regarding layout and style when writing a research report.

As another level of evaluation, it is useful, before you finish the activity, to note down:

(a) what you learned from doing the activity,
(b) how you will use what you learned,
(c) how what you have learned relates to what you have read, and
(d) what you need to learn next.

- Use short sentences.
- Do not use long words when simpler ones would do.
- Keep jargon and technical terms to a minimum.
- Do not use long paragraphs. If you plan your writing, you can divide up what you have to say into manageable 'chunks'.
- Use headings to guide the reader.
- Remember *who* you are writing for: the audience for your writing may dictate the style.
- Edit your work frequently. Cut out all unnecessary words and phrases. Avoid 'padding'.
- Be prepared to make several drafts of your report.
- Show your work *(a)* to your supervisor, for comments and *(b)* to an 'outsider', who has nothing to do with the field. Listen to the latter's comments carefully!

If necessary, consult a style manual to help you to present your findings and to learn to use the appropriate style for writing research reports. Examples of such style manuals include:

CBE Style Manual, 5th edn, Council of Biology Editors, Bethesda, Maryland.

Turabian, K.L. (1973) *A Manual For Writers of Term Papers, Theses and Dissertations*, 4th edn, University of Chicago Press, Chicago.

Consider reading the following 'classics' on how to write well:

Strunk, W. Jr and White, E.B. (1972) *The Elements of Style*, 2nd edn, Macmillan, New York.

Gowers, E. (revised by B. Fraser) (1977) *The Complete Plain Words*, 2nd edn, Penguin, Harmondsworth.

Working with a Computer

Many people, nowadays, write directly to a computer screen, using a word processing package. This is a particularly economical way of using your time and is much better than writing longhand and then transferring your work to the computer. Here are some points about the use of a word processor and writing a research report:

- Get to know your computer well. If it is a *personal computer* (IBM compatible) you will need to decide whether to use *DOS programs* or *Windows* programs. If you are new to computing, if you want to use more than one program at a time and if you want to be able to transfer data quickly and easily between programs, then *Windows* programs are generally the best ones to use. On the other hand, *Windows* programs call for a speedy processing chip (386 or better), lots of memory (RAM) and a large hard disk.

- Try to learn *all* of the functions of your word processor. Many people use word processors as glorified typewriters but this is to miss the point. Used fully, a word processor can help you to check your spelling and grammar, count your words, enable you to transfer data from one part of a document to another, compile an index for your report, and enable you to produce a professional-looking document.
- Divide your report up into small sections and open up a new file for each section. Many word processors have a function that allow you to quickly and easily draw together a number of related files into a 'master-file' that allows you to view the whole of your document as one piece of work.
- Save your work regularly and make back-ups of your work to floppy disks. On the other hand, also make full use of your hard disk. Some people get into the odd habit of working from floppy disks and using the hard disk only for storing programs. This, again, is to miss the point of working with computers. A hard disk is much faster than floppies.
- Don't make *lots* of 'hard copies' of your work (a hard copy is a printed one). On the other hand, make one such copy just before you print out your *final* report and edit it. It is often easy to miss minor errors when you are reading text on the computer monitor.
- Get to know the local 'computer expert'. Don't panic if things go wrong. Stop what you are doing and call the expert. You can often *undelete* files that you think you have lost but *only* if you don't reuse the computer after you have made a major error.
- Find out what computing facilities are available in your college and make full use of them. Apply to go on software training courses if they are available. On the other hand, do not feel that you have to learn to *program* with a computer. These days, not many users have to develop programming skills but *all* have to learn to use the software that is available.

Further Reading

Burnard, P. (1993) *Personal Computing for Health Professionals*, Chapman & Hall, London.

Hannah, K.J. (1987) 'Uses for computers in nursing research', *Recent Advances in Nursing*, **17**, 186–202.

Morse, J.M. and Morse, R.M. (1989) 'QUAL: a mainframe program for qualitative data analysis', *Nursing Research*, **38** (3) 188–9.

Rose, D. and Sullivan, O. (1993) *Introducing Data Analysis for Social Scientists*, Open University Press, Milton Keynes.

10.3 Writing for Publication

By the end of this section you will have discovered:

- How to prepare your work for publication;
- How to acquire guidelines for publication.

Opportunities for Publication

Your report may be considered for publication by a number of organisations. Some opportunities for publishing your work include:

- As a journal article
- As a 'short report' in a journal of abstracts
- As a chapter in a book
- As a book
- As a monograph published by your college, school or university department
- As a published conference paper
- As a local report in your organisation.

Reasons for Publishing Research Reports

Strauss and Corbin, in a discussion about writing and publishing parts of these and monographs, offer the following points about publishing research:

1. . . . researchers may decide to publish papers even relatively early during the research process. They may do this for different reasons. For instance, to present preliminary findings, or to satisfy or impress sponsors, or because they have interesting materials bearing on side issues that can easily be written up now but might not get written at a later more hectic time.
2. Sometimes researchers write papers because they feel either obligated to publish on a given topic or because they are pressured to do so. Of course this motivation will also affect what and how a researcher writes.
3. Researchers may also be invited to contribute papers to special issues of journals or edited volumes, because they are known to be researching in given areas. They may also be urged or tempted to convert verbal presentations into papers, because listeners have responded well to them.
4. Another condition that can affect the writing of a paper is the existence of a deadline for getting the finished product to an editor. For some researchers this can act as a stimulus, while others of course are daunted by any deadline.

5. The number of pages allowed by the editor also affects whether a paper will be written – at least for this particular publication – and what will be written and how.
6. Unless invited by an editor, there is the important decision to be made about which particular journal should be elected as a potential outlet for a given paper. Journals and papers have to be matched, otherwise time is wasted in its rejection, or worse yet the paper is accepted but for an inappropriate or insufficiently appreciative audience. (Strauss and Corbin, 1990)

Reporting Your Findings to Respondents and Others

There are various ways that others can learn of your research. Some methods of disseminating your findings include:

- Discussion groups in the school of nursing;
- Submitting an abstract to a conference;
- Inviting respondents to a study day;
- Through a local research interest group;
- Local publications within the school, college or university.

Exercise 10.3

Aim of the exercise: To explore research reports that have been published

Planning stage: You can do this exercise on your own or in the company of a small group of colleagues, friends or students. Allow yourself plenty of time to complete the exercise and make notes of what you do, as you go. If you work with friends or colleagues, decide whether you will all carry out similar tasks or you will divide up the work between you.

Equipment/resources required: Notebook, pen and access to a nursing library.

What to do: Obtain the following research reports (books and journals), from the library. Read them and make notes under the following headings:

- Was the report interesting?
- Was the report relevant: did it have implications for practice or for further research?

- Did the writer's style keep your attention or was it difficult to finish reading the paper or book?
- Would you have read it by choice?
- Would it have wide appeal?

Now study the following books on writing for publication:

- Burnard, P. (1992) *Writing for Health Professionals*, Chapman & Hall, London.
- O'Connor, M. (1978) *Editing Scientific Books and Journals*, Pitman Medical, London,
- Sternberg, R.J. (1988) *The Psychologist's Companion: A Guide to Writing Scientific Papers for Students and Researchers*, Cambridge University Press, Cambridge.
- Starr, A.D. (1988) *Science Writing for Beginners*, Blackwell, Oxford.

Evaluation: Discuss your findings with your colleagues and draw out the ingredients of a good published report. Remember that, from the publisher's point of view, the main question is 'Will this article or book *sell*?' Note that this raises different evaluation criteria from those that apply to evaluating research reports that are not for publication. A written report may be excellent but it will not get published if it does not help to sell the book or journal. But . . . keep trying! The value to yourself and others of having a report published is worth the effort.

Submitting Work for Consideration for Publication

Getting your report published may be an important aspect of the sharing and development of knowledge. Whilst you may have to wait a while before you see your work published, and there can be no guarantee that your work will be accepted, the following guidelines may help to speed up the process:

- Approach one journal with the *idea* of your report. This allows you and the publisher to know whether or not there is a likelihood of acceptance for publication.
- Only submit to one journal at a time. You could be embarrassed if two journals accepted your work! It is also illegal to publish the same piece of work in two journals, without permission from the first publisher.
- Ask a journal's editor for a copy of their 'Advice to Authors'. Follow their advice to the letter. Sometimes this information is contained inside the back page of the journal itself.

- Prepare only blemish-free copies. A scruffy manuscript is unlikely to impress editors.
- Be prepared for a journal to reject your work. Some will write back with details of how your work could be modified. Others won't. If you do get advice on how to revise your work, follow that advice carefully. The editor always knows best!
- Keep a copy of anything you submit for publication and note the date on which you send work off to journals.

Conclusion

You have now completed your research! Now you can consider your next move: will you do more research, further study ... another course? Your work has stopped for the moment but, if you are to continue your education as a nurse, you need to consider the next step. We hope that you have enjoyed working through this book and through the process of research. Good luck!

Learning Check

If You are Working on Your Own

Read through the notes that you have kept whilst completing the exercises in this chapter and consider the following questions:

- What new knowledge have I gained?
- What new skills have I developed?
- How has my thinking about research changed?
- What do I need to do now?

Check that you have made reference cards for any new references that you have found whilst working on the exercises in this chapter.

If You are Working in a Small Group

Pair off and nominate one of you as A and one of you as B. For five minutes, A talks to B about what she has learned and A listens. This should *not* be a conversation: B's only role is to listen. After five minutes, roles are reversed and B talks to A about what she has learned and A listens. After the second five minutes, re-form into a group a discuss the experience.

If You are a Tutor and/or Facilitator

- Use the above pairs exercise with the group you are working with.
- Hold two 'rounds' in which each person in turn says *(a)* what she liked least about doing the activities and *(b)* what she liked most about doing the activities

Compendium of Useful Information

In this compendium you will find a whole host of ideas and pointers to further information which will help any nurse involved in research. The compendium does not pretend to be exhaustive but it does point you in the right direction for a successful project.

How to Quote References in Research Reports

Clear and accurate references should always be offered in a research report. These references allow other readers to:

- verify what you write;
- develop your ideas further;
- identify other sources or reading.

It is important that you list only publications that you have actually read so that your use of references is accurate. It is also important that you record your references accurately and systematically. Various methods of referencing are available but perhaps the most frequently used method is known as the Harvard method.

Attention to the details of this system is important and it is vital that you do not mix two sorts of referencing systems together! Learn this one and use it accurately. Once learned, the method of referencing can be used for nearly all essays, papers and submissions to journals.

The Harvard Referencing System

In the text you refer to references by surname only and year of publication, as illustrated in the following passage.

Although first prepared by Benedikt (1879), its structure was not confirmed until much later (Osborn and Jay, 1955). Fox, Keenan and Trueside (1983) have recently shown that it is a good chlorinating agent.

Note that when you reference in this way, you do not refer to the title of the book or article in the text. This is listed in a separate section of your report.

If you quote directly from a reference and you only want to quote a few words, you do so as follows:

Counselling has been described as the process of 'exploring the other person's world' (Black, 1986).

If you quote direct from a reference and you want to quote a slightly longer piece, you do so as follows:

'Empathy is the intimate process of coming to view the world as the other persons's frame of reference' (Black, 1986, pp. 22–3).

If you want to use a quotation that has already been used by another writer, you do so as follows:

'Empathy cannot be taught, it can only be learned through direct personal experience' (Brown, cited by White, 1987, p. 22).

In the reference list, you then list *White's* book – the one that contained the quotation. Wherever possible, you should avoid quoting from secondary sources. Try to go back to the original.

If you want to quote from a chapter by one author, that is contained in a book edited by another, you do so as follows:

Interpersonal skills may be taught in a variety of settings. As one writer points out: 'Interpersonal skills training is often associated with psychiatric nursing. It is just as vital in general nursing, health visiting and district nursing' (Jones, 1987, p. 34)

In the reference list, the chapter is entered as follows:

Jones, D. (1987) 'Teaching Interpersonal Skills', in D. Brown (ed.), <u>A Handbook of Training Methods for Nurses</u>, Heinemann, London.

Note, particularly, the style of layout of this reference and the underlining procedure. For further details of this, see below.

There are certain specific points to be made about using direct quotes:

- only use quotations that add significantly to your work;
- when you use a direct quotation, keep it short and indent the paragraph;
- after the quotation and in brackets, identify the author, date of publication and page number(s).

At the end of your paper you should include a list of references. This should be in alphabetical order of authors' surnames and is subject to certain conventions. If you are referencing a book in your list, it should appear as in the following example:

Burnard, P. (1990) Learning Human Skills: A Guide for Nurses, 2nd edition, Butterworth-Heinemann, Oxford.

A book is identified by the following details:

- author
- date of publication
- title
- publisher
- place of publication.

If you are referencing a journal article it should appear as follows:

Riebel, L. (1984) 'A Homeopathic Model of Psychotherapy', Journal of Humanistic Psychology, vol. 24, no. 2, 9–14.

A journal article is identified by the following details:

- author
- date of publication
- title of the article
- name of the journal
- volume number
- edition number
- page range.

Note an important difference between referencing books and articles. In the case of a book, the title is underlined, but in the case of an article, the name of the *journal* is underlined.

Reference lists differ from bibliographies, which provide a further list of books and journals that the writer has found of interest. Normally, a research report will contain only a reference list.

Computer Programs

Computer programs are always being improved. This list offers an idea of the range of programs available.

Computer programs fall into categories:

- word processing
- databases
- spreadsheet
- integrated programs
- statistical programs.

Word processors are the programs that help you to write your report. A good word-processing package will include many of the following facilities:

- word counting
- spelling check
- movement of text
- ability to edit two documents concurrently
- fast movement through text.

Examples of word-processing programs are:

- Word for Windows
- WordPerfect for Windows
- Ami Pro
- LetterPerfect
- Locoscript.

Databases allow you to store information. You may use such a program to store all the references that you collect or to store the research data that you have accumulated. A good database program will include many of the following facilities:

- fast movement through entries;
- alphabetical sorting;
- flexibility
- ability to import and export data.

Examples of database programs are:

- Pardox for Windows
- Access
- Agenda

160

- Superbase
- Info Select.

Spreadsheets allow you to draw large 'grids' and tables to allow you to think about and analyse your data. A good spreadsheet program will include many of the following facilities:

- flexibility
- ability to import data
- simple word processing
- mathematical and statistical ability
- graphics.

Examples of spreadsheet programs are:

- Excel for Windows
- Lotus 123
- PlanPerfect
- Quattro Pro for Windows.

Integrated programs incorporate word processing, database and spreadsheet functions. An integrated program allows you to transfer data quickly from one element of the program to another. The drawbacks of such programs are that they are often expensive to buy and the individual elements of the program may not be so easy to use as separate programs. A good integrated program will include many of the following facilities:

- easy transfer of data
- ease of use
- good graphics.

Examples of integrated programs are:

- CA Office
- Lotus Works
- Borland Office
- Works for Windows.

Statistical packages are those programs that help you with the analysis of data. Many spreadsheet programs are also able to do statistical calculations.
Examples of statistical packages are:

- SPSS for Windows
- C-Stat for Windows
- Unistat for Windows.

Other programs are available to help you prepare, analyse and present your data. Programs that you may want to consider are those concerned with:

- analysing data;
- creating an index;
- creating graphics;
- desktop publishing;
- expert systems;
- money management;
- teaching.

Useful introductory texts for computing include:

Burnard, P. (1993) *Personal Computing for Health Professionals*, Chapman & Hall, London.
Blease, D. (1986) *Evaluating Educational Software*, Croom Helm, London.
Proter, P. (1988) *Nurses and Computers*, Croom Helm, London.
Rowntree, G. (ed.) (1987) *Fundamentals of Computing*, NCC Publications, Manchester.

Literature Resources

It is important that your literature search is as comprehensive as possible. Here is a list of possible sources of information.

- Books
- Colleagues
- Leaflets
- Journals
- Computer searches
- Unpublished reports
- Papers
- Supervisors
- Posters
- Special libraries
- Radio or TV
- Handouts
- RCN (Royal College of Nursing)
- Teletext

Ethical Codes

Ethical issues frequently arise when conducting research. One way of thinking about ethical dilemmas is to consult a code of conduct. In 1984, the United Kingdom Central Council for Nursing, Midwifery and Health Visiting produced the following Code of Professional Conduct.

Each registered nurse, midwife and health visitor shall act, at all times, in such a manner as to justify public trust and confidence, to uphold and enhance the good standing and reputation of the profession, to serve the interests of society, and above all to safeguard the interests of society, and above all to safeguard the interests of individual patients and client.

Each registered nurse, midwife and health visitor is accountable for his or her practice and, in the exercise of professional accountability shall:

1. Act always in such a way as to promote and safeguard the well being and interests of patients/clients.
2. Ensure that no action or omission on his/her part or within his/her sphere of influence is detrimental to the condition of safety of patients/clients.
3. Take every reasonable opportunity to maintain professional knowledge and competence.
4. Acknowledge any limitations of competence and refuse in such cases to accept delegated functions without first having received instruction in regard to those functions and having been assessed as competent.
5. Work in a collaborative and co-operative manner with other health care professionals and recognise and respect their particular contributions within the health care team.
6. Take account of the customs, values and spiritual beliefs of patients/clients.
7. Make known to an appropriate person or authority any conscientious objections which may be relevant to professional practice.
8. Avoid any abuse of privileged relationship which exists with patients/clients and of the privileged access allowed to their property, residence or workman.
9. Respect confidential information obtained in the course of professional practice and refrain from disclosing such information without the consent of the patient/client, or a person entitled to act on his/her behalf, except where disclosure is required by law or by the order of a court or is necessary in the public interest.
10. Have regard to the environment of care and its physical, psychological and social effects on patients/clients, and also to the adequacy of resources, and make known to appropriate persons or authorities any

circumstances which could place patients/clients in jeopardy or which militate against safe standards of practice.

11. Have regard to the workload of and the pressures on professional colleagues and subordinates and take appropriate action if these are seen to be such to constitute abuse of the individual practitioner and/ or to jeopardise safe standards of practice.

12. In the context of the individual's own knowledge, experience, and sphere of authority, assist peers and subordinates to develop professional competence in accordance with their needs.

13. Refuse to accept any gift, favour or hospitality which might be interpreted as seeking to exert undue influence to obtain preferential consideration.

14. Avoid the use of professional qualifications in the promotion of commercial products in order not to compromise the independence of professional judgement on which patients/clients rely.

Nurses, too, are often required to take into account medical decisions when planning their research. In 1964, guidelines for doctors working in clinical research were laid down by the World Medical Assembly. The Declaration of Helsinki reads as follows:

In the treatment of the sick person, the doctor must be free to use a new therapeutic measure if, in his judgement, it offers hope of saving life, re-establishing health, or alleviating suffering. If at all possible, consistent with patient psychology, the doctor should obtain the patient's freely given consent after the patient has been given a full explanation. In case of legal incapacity, consent should be procured from the legal guardian; in case of physical incapacity, the permission of the legal guardian replaces that of the patient.

The doctor can combine clinical research with professional care, the objective being the acquisition of new medical knowledge, only to the extent that clinical research is justified by its therapeutic value for the patient.

In the purely scientific application of clinical research carried out on a human being, it is the duty of the doctor to remain the protector of life and health of that person on whom clinical research is being carried out.

The nature, the purpose, and the risk of clinical research must be explained to the subject by the doctor.

Clinical research on a human being cannot be undertaken without his free consent, after he has been fully informed; if he is legally incompetent, the consent of the legal guardian should be procured.

The subject of clinical research should be in such a mental, physical and legal state as to be able to exercise fully his power of choice.

Consent should, as a rule, be obtained in writing. However, the responsibility for clinical research always remains with the research worker; it never falls on the subject even after consent is obtained.

The investigator must respect the right of each individual to safeguard his personal integrity, especially if the subject is in a dependent relationship to the investigator.

At any time during the course of clinical research, the subject or his guardian should be free to withdraw permission for research to be continued. The investigator or the investigating team should discontinue the research if, in his or their judgment it may, if continued, be harmful to the individual.

References

Declaration of Helsinki: *Recommendations Guiding Doctors in Clinical Research, Adopted by the 18th World Medical Assembly, Helsinki, Finland,* 1964.

RCN (1977) *Ethics Related to Research in Nursing,* Royal College of Nursing, London.

UKCC (1984) *Code of Professional Conduct for the Nurse, Midwife and Health Visitor,* 2nd edn, United Kingdom Central Council for Nursing, Midwifery and Health Visiting, London.

List of Nursing Journals

Advances in Nursing Science
American Journal of Nursing
Applied Nursing Research
Australian Journal of Advanced Nursing
Archives of Psychiatric Nursing
British Journal of Nursing
Critical Care Nurse
Clinical Care Specialist
Gynaecological and Neonatal Nursing
Health Education Journal
Health Visitor

Journal of District Nursing
Journal of Clinical Nursing
Journal of Medical Ethics
Maternal-Child Nursing Journal
Midwifery
Nurse Education Today
Nursing
Nursing Research
Nursing Clinics of North America
Nursing Times
Nursing Outlook
Nursing Standard
Professional Nurse

Intensive Care Nursing
International Journal of Nursing
   Studies
Issues in Mental Health Nursing
Journal of Obstetrics
Journal of Psychiatric Nursing
Journal of Nursing Education
Journal of Advanced Nursing

Recent Advances in Nursing
Research in Nursing and Health
Scholarly Inquiry for Nursing
Senior Nurse
Surgical Nurse
Western Journal of Nursing
Research

Lists of Bibliographies, Indexes and Abstracts

Abstracts, Information for Education
American Psychological Association
Bibliographic Index, Wilson
British National Bibliography
British Books in Print, Whitaker
British Library Bibliographic Services Division
British Humanities Index, Wilson
British Library Services
Child Development Abstracts
Current Literature on Health Services, Department of Health
Current Index to Journals in Education, ERIC
Current Index to Journals in Education, Macmillan
Education Index, Wilson
Hospital Abstracts, Her Majesty's Stationery Office (HMSO)
Index to Theses, ASLIB
Indexes, Wilson
Institute for Scientific Information
International Nursing Index
National Library of Medicine
Nursing Research Abstracts
Nursing Bibliography, RCN
Psychological Abstracts
Research into Higher Education
Resources in Education, ERIC
Social Trends, HMSO
Social Sciences Citation Index
Social Services Abstracts, Department of Social Services (DSS)
Society for Research into Higher Education
Sociology of Education
Subject Guide to Books in Print
Technical Education Abstracts
The British Education Index

Tests, Scales and Other Instruments for Data Collection

Andrulis, R.A. (1977) *A Source Book of Tests and Measures of Human Behaviour* Charles C. Thomas, Springfield, Illinois.

Antonak, R.F. and Livneh, H. (1988) *The Measurement of Attitudes toward People with Disabilities: Methods, Psychometrics and Scales*, Charles C. Thomas, Springfield, Illinois.

Beere, C.A. (1979) *Women and Women's Issues: A Handbook of Tests and Measurements*, Jossey Bass, San Francisco, California.

Bonjean, C.M., Hill, R.J. and McLemore, S.D. (1967) *Sociological Measurement: An Inventory of Scales and Indices*, Chandler Publishing, San Francisco, California.

Bower, J.D., Ackerman, P.G. and Toro, G. (1974) *Clinical Laboratory Methods*, 8th edn, C.V. Mosby, St Louis.

Bowling, A. (1991) *Measuring Health: A Review of Quality of Life Measurement Scales*, Open University Press, Milton Keynes.

Catell, R.B. and Warburton, F. (1976) *Objective Personality and Motivation Tests: A Theoretical Introduction and Practical Compendium*, University of Illinois Press, Urbana.

Chun, Ki-Taek, Cobb, S. and French, J.R. (1975) *Measures for Psychological Assessment: A Guide to 3,000 Original Sources and Their Applications*, Institute for Social Research, Ann Arbor, Michigan.

Ciminero, A.R., Calhoun, K.S. and Adams. H.E. (eds) (1977) *Handbook of Behavioural Assessment*, Wiley, New York.

Comrey, A.L., Backer, T.E. and Glaser, E.M. (1973) *A Source Book for Mental Health Measures*, Human Interaction Research Institute, Los Angeles, California.

Cromwell, L., Webell, F.J. and Pfeiffer, E.A. (1980) *Biomedical Instrumentation and Measurements*, 2nd edn, Prentice-Hall, Engelwood Cliffs, New Jersey.

Ferris, C. (1980) *A Guide to Medical Laboratory Instruments*, Little, Brown, Boston.

Geddes, L.A. and Baker, L.E. (1975) *Principles of Applied Biomedical Instrumentation*, Wiley, New York.

General Practice Research Unit (1969) *General Health Questionnaire*, NFER-Nelson Publishing, Windsor, Berks.

Goldman, B.A. and Saunders, J.L. (1974) *Directory of Unpublished Experimental Measures: Vol I*, Behavioral Publications, New York.

Goldman, B.A. and Saunders, J.L. (1978) *Directory of Unpublished Experimental Measures: Vol II*, Behavioral Publications, New York.

Haussmann, R.K.D., Hegyvary, S.T. and Newman, J.F. (1976) *The Rush-Medicus-Monitoring Methodology: Monitoring Quality of Nursing Care, Part 2 – Assessment and Study of Correlates*, DHEW Publication HRA

167

76-7, US Government Printing Office, Washington DC.

Henerson, M.E., Morris, L.L. and Fitz-Gibbon, C.T. (1978) *How To Measure Attitudes*, Sage, London.

Jacox, A.K. Prescott, P.A., Collar, K. and Goodwin, L.D. (1981) *The Nurse Practitioner Rating Form: A Primary Care Process Measure*, Nursing Resources, Wakefield, Massachusetts.

Johnson, O.G. (1976) *Tests and Measurements in Child Development, Handbook II, Vols 1 and 2*, Jossey Bass, San Francisco, California.

Johnson, O.G. and Commarito, J.W. (1971) *Tests and Measurements in Child Development, Handbook I*, Jossey Bass, San Francisco, California.

Karoly, P. (ed.) (1985) *Measurement Strategies in Health Psychology*, Wiley, New York.

Lake, D.G., Miles, M.B. and Earle, R.B. (1973) *Measuring Behavior*, Teachers' College Press, New York.

Lyerly, S. (1973) *Handbook of Psychiatric Rating Scales*, 2nd edn, National Institutes of Mental Health, Rockville, Maryland.

McDowell, I. and Newell, C. (1987) *Measuring Health: A Guide to Rating Scales and Questionnaires*, Oxford University Press, New York.

Miller, D.C. (1991) *Handbook of Research Design and Social Measurement*, 5th edn, David McKay, New York.

Pfeiffer, W.J., Heslen, R. and Jones, J.E. (1976) *Instrumentation in Human Relations Training*, 2nd edn, University Associates, La Jolla, California.

Phaneuf, M.C. (1976) *The Nursing Audit: Self-Regulation of Nursing Practice*, Appleton-Century-Crofts, New York.

Price, J.L. (1972) *Handbook of Organisational Measurement*, D.C. Heath, Lexington, Massachusetts.

Reeder, L.G., Ramacher, L. and Gorelnik, S. (1976) *Handbook of Scales and Indices of Health Behavior*, Goodyear, Pacific Palisades, California.

Robinson, J.P., Athanasiou, R. and Head, K.B. (1969) *Measures of Occupational Attitudes and Occupational Characteristics*, Institute for Social Research, University of Michigan, Ann Arbor, Michigan.

Robinson, J.P. and Shaver, P.R. (1973) *Measures of Social Psychological Attitudes*, Institute for Social Research, University of Michigan, Ann Arbor, Michigan.

Shaw, M.E. and Wright, J.M. (1967) *Scales for the Measurement of Attitudes*, McGraw-Hill, New York.

Strauss, M.A. and Brown, B.W. (1978) *Family Measurement Techniques – Abstracts of Published Instruments 1935–1974*, rev. edn, University of Minnesota Press, Minneapolis.

Wandelt, A. and Ager, J. (1975) *Quality Patient Care Scale (Qualpacs)*, Appleton-Century-Crofts, New York.

Wandelt, A. and Stewart, D.S. (1975) *Slater Nursing Competencies Rating Scale*, Appleton-Century-Crofts, New York.

Ward, M.J. and Felter, M.E. (1979) *Instruments for Use in Nursing Educa-*

tion Research, Western Interstate Commission for Higher Education, Boulder, Colorado.

Weiss, M. (1973) *Biomedical Instrumentation*, Chilton Book Co., Philadelphia.

Useful Addresses and Sources of Information

Department of Health Library
Alexander Fleming House
London
SE1 6BY

English National Board for Nursing, Midwifery and Health Visiting
Victory House
170 Tottenham Court Road
London
W1P OHA

English National Board for Nursing, Midwifery and Health Visiting
Learning Resources Unit
Chantrey House
789 Chesterfield Road
Sheffield
S8 OSF

King's Fund Centre Library
126 Albert Street
London
NW1 7NF

Royal College of Nursing Library
20 Cavendish Square
London
W1M OAB
(The Royal College of Nursing Library also houses the Steinberg Collection
of United Kingdom and North American Nursing Theses and Dissertations.)

United Kingdom Central Council for Nursing, Midwifery and Health Visiting
23 Portland Place
London
W1N 3AF

Bibliography

References

Gilbert, G. (ed.) (1993) *Researching Social Life*, Sage, London.

Godefroy, C.H. and Clark, J. (1939) *The Complete Time Management System*, Piatkus, London.

Hammersley, M. (1992) *What's Wrong with Ethnography?*, Routledge, London.

Kelly, G.A. (1955) *The Psychology of Personal Constructs*, 2 vols, Norton, New York.

Lewin, K. (1946) 'Action Research and Minority Problems', *Journal of Social Issues*, 2 34–46.

Linstone, H.A. and M. (ed) (1975) *The Delphi Method: Technique and Application'*, Addison-Wesley, Reading, Mass.

May, T. (1993) *Social Research: Issues, Method and Process*, Open University, Milton Keynes.

Oppenheim, A.N. (1992) *Questionnaire Design, Interviewing and Altitude Measurement*, 2nd edn, Printer Press, London.

Robson, C. (1993) *Real World Research*, Blackwell.Oxford.

SERC (1983) *Research Student and Supervisor: An Approach to Good Supervisory Practice*. Issued by SERC, Polaris House, North Star Avenue, Swindon, SN2 1ET.

Sommer, R. and Sommer, B.B. (1991) *A Practical Guide to Behavioural Research: Tools and Techniques*, Oxford University Press, New York.

Stephenson, W. (1953) *The Study of Behaviour: Q. Technique and its Methodology*, University of Chicago Press, Chicago.

Strauss, A. and Carbin, J. (1990) *Basics of Qualitative Research*, Sage, London.

Tajfel, H. and Frazer, C. (eds) (1978) *Introducing Social Psychology*, Penguin, Harmondsworth.

Recommended Further Reading

Abrahams, P. (1982) *Historical Sociology*, Open Books, Shepton Mallet.

Agar, M. (1986) *Speaking of Ethnography*, Sage, Beverly Hills, California.

170

Agar, M. (1980) *The Professional Stranger. An Informal Introduction to Ethnography*, Academic Press, New York.

Altman, D.G., Gore, S.M., Gardner, M.J. and Pocock, S.J. (1983) 'Statistical Guidelines for Contributors to Medical Journals', *British Medical Journal*, **286**, 1489–93.

Anastasi, A. (1988) *Psychological Testing*, 6th edn, Macmillan, New York.

Ashworth, P.D. (1987) *Adequacy of Description: The Validity of Qualitative Findings*, Sheffield Papers in Education Management 67, Sheffield City Polytechnic.

Ashworth, P.D., Giorgi, A. and de Koning, A.J.J. (eds) (1986) *Qualitative Research in Psychology: Proceedings of the International Association for Qualitative Research*, Duquesne University Press, Pittsburgh, Pennsylvania.

Atkinson, P. (1981) *The Clinical Experience*, Gower, Farnborough, Hampshire.

Babbie, E. (1983) *The Practice of Social Research*, 3rd edn, Wadsworth, Belmont, California.

Ball, M.J. and Hannah, K.J. (1984) *Using Computers in Nursing*, Reston Publishing, Reston.

Ball, S.J. (1983) 'Case Study Research in Education – Some Notes and Problems' in M. Hammersley (ed.) *The Ethnography of Schooling Methodological Issues*, Nafferton Books, Driffield, Humberside.

Bannister, D., and Mair, J.M.M. (1968) *The Evaluation of Personal Constructs*, Academic Press, London.

Barhyte, D. and Bacon, L.D. (1985) 'Approaches to cleaning data sets: a technical comment', *Nursing Research*, **34**, 62–4.

Barker, P. (1991) 'Questionnaire' in D.F.S. Cormack (ed.) *The Research Process in Nursing*, 2nd edn. Blackwell, Oxford, pp. 215–27.

Bayliss, D. (1983) 'Statistics for nurses', *Nursing Times*, **79**, 47–50.

Bell, C. and Newby, H. (eds) (1977) *Doing Sociological Research*, Allen & Unwin, London.

Bell, R.C. (1988) 'Theory-appropriate analysis of repertory grid data', *International Journal of Personal Construct Psychology*, **1**, 101–18.

Belson, W.A. (1981) *The Design and Understanding of Survey Questions*, Gower, Aldershot.

Berelson, B. (1952) *Content Analysis in Communication Research*, The Free Press, Glencoe, Illinois.

Berelson, B. (1971) *Content Analysis in Communication Research*, Free Press, New York.

Berg, B.L. (1989) *Qualitative Research Methods for the Social Sciences*, Allyn & Bacon, Boston.

Borzak, L. (ed.) (1981) *Field Study: A Sourcebook for Experimental Learning*, Sage, Beverly Hills, California.

Brenner, M. (1985) 'Intensive interviewing' in M. Brenner, J. Brown and D. Canter (eds) *The Research Interview: Uses and Approaches*, Academic Press, London, pp. 147–62.

Brenner, M., Brown, J. and Canter, D. (eds) (1985) *The Research Interview: Uses and Approaches*; Academic Press, London.

Brinberg, D. and McGrath, J.E. (1985) *Validity and the Research Process*, Sage, Beverly Hills, California.

British Museum, *General Catalogue of Printed Books*, British Museum, London.

British Psychological Society (1978) *Statement on Ethical Principles for Research with Human Subjects*, BPS, Leicester.

British Standards Institute (1978) *Recommendations for Citing Publications by Bibliographic References*, London.

Brooking, J. (ed.) (1986) *Psychiatric Nursing Research*, Wiley, Chichester.

Bryman, A. (1984) 'The debate about quantitative and qualitative research: a question of method or epistemology?' *British Journal of Sociology*, **35** 65–92.

Burcham, W.E. and Rutherford, R.J.D. (eds) (1987) *Writing Application for Research Grants*, 2nd edn, Educational Development Advisory Committee, Occasional Publications No. 3, University of Birmingham.

Cahoon, M.C. (ed.) (1987) *Research Methodology*, Recent Advances in Nursing Series, 17, Churchill Livingstone, Edinburgh.

Calnan, J. (1976) *One Way to Do Research: The A–Z for Those who Must*, Heinemann, London.

Canter, D. (ed.) (1985) *Facet Theory: Approaches to Social Research*, Springer-Verlag, New York.

Canter, D., Brown, J., and Groat, L. (1985) 'A multiple sorting procedure for studying conceptual systems' in M. Brenner, J. Brown and D. Canter (eds) (1985) *The Research Interview: Uses and Approaches*, Academic Press, London, pp. 79–114.

Chenitz, W.C. and Swanson, J.M. (1986) *From Practice to Grounded Theory: Qualitative Research in Nursing*, Addison Wesley, Menlo Park, New York.

Clegg, F. (1990) *Simple Statistics: A Course Guide for the Social Sciences*, Cambridge University Press, Cambridge.

Converse, J.M. and Presser, S. (1986) *Survey Questions. Handcrafting the Standardised Questionnaire*, Sage, London.

Coolican, H. (1990) *Research Methods and Statistics in Psychology*, Hodder & Stoughton, London.

Costigan, J., Humphrey, J., & Murphy, C. (1987) 'Attempted suicide: a personal construct psychology exploration', *Australian Journal of Advanced Nursing*, **4** (2) 39–50.

Cronbach, L.J. (1984) *Essentials of Psychological Testing*, 4th edn, Harper & Row, New York.

Darling, V.H. and Rogers J. (1986) *Research for Practising Nurses*, Macmillan, Basingstoke.

Davis, A.J. (1985) 'Ethical Issues in Nursing Research', *Western Journal of Nursing Research*, **7**, 125–6.

Davis, B.D. (1983) *Research into Nurse Education*, Croom Helm, London.

Deising, P, (1971) *Patterns of Discovery in the Social Sciences*, Aldine, New York.

Dempsey, P.A. and Dempsey, A.D. (1986) *The Research Process in Nursing*, Jones & Bartlett, Boston, Massachusetts.

Dennis, K.E. (1986) 'Q methodology: relevance and application to nursing research', *Advances in Nursing Science*, **8**, 6–17.

Denzin, N.K. (1973) *The Research Act: A Theoretical Introduction to Sociological Methods*, Aldine, New York.

Denzin, N.M. (1978) *Sociological Methods: A Sourcebook*, 2nd edn, McGraw-Hill, New York.

De Vaus, D.A. (1991) *Surveys in Social Research*, 3rd edn, George Allen & Unwin, London.

DeVellis, B.N., Adams. J.L. and De Vellis, R.F. (1984) 'Effects of information on patient stereotyping, *Research in Nursing and Health*, **7**, 237–44.

Dilman, D. (1978) *Mail and Telephone Surveys: The Total Design Method*, Wiley, New York.

Dissertation Abstracts International, Ann Arbor, Michigan.

Douglas, J. (1976) *Investigative Social Research*, Sage, Beverly Hills, California.

Dowrick, P. and Briggs, S.J. (eds) (1983) *Using Video: Psychological and Social Applications*, Wiley, New York.

Duffy, M.E. (1985) 'Designing nursing research: the qualitative–quantitative debate', *Journal of Advanced Nursing*, **10**, 225–31.

Epting, F. (1984) *Personal Construct Counselling and Psychotherapy*, Wiley, Chichester.

Feyerbend, P. (1978) *Against Method*, Varo, London.

Fielding, N.G. and Fielding, J.L. (1985) *Linking Data*, Sage, Beverly Hills, California.

Filstead, W.J. (1970) *Qualitative Methodology: Firsthand Involvement with the Social World*. Rand McNally, Chicago.

Fink, A. and Kosekoff, J. (1985) *How to Conduct Surveys: A Step-by-Step Guide*, Sage, Beverly Hills, California.

Fox, D.J. (1982) *Fundamentals of Research in Nursing*, 4th edn, Appleton-Century-Crofts, Norwalk, New Jersey.

Fransella, F. and Bannister, D. (1977) *A Manual for Repertory Grid Technique*, Academic Press, London.

Gardner, G. (1978) *Social Surveys for Social Planners*, Open University Press, Milton Keynes.

George, T.B. (1982) 'Development of the self-concept of nurse in nursing students', *Research in Nursing and Health*, **5**, 191–7.

Glaser, B.G. (1978) *Theoretical Sensitivity: Advances in the Methodology of Grounded Theory*, Sociology Press, Mill Valley, California.

Godsmith, J.W. (1981) 'Methodological considerations in using videotape to establish rater reliability', *Nursing Research*, **30** 124–7.

Goffman, E. (1971) *The Presentation of Self in Everyday Life*, Harmondsworth, Penguin.

Goodwin, L. and Goodwin, W. (1984) 'Qualitative vs quantitative research or qualitative and quantitative research?'; *Nursing Research*, **33** 378–80.

Groat, L. (1982) 'Meaning in post-modern architecture: an examination using the multiple sorting task', *Journal of Environmental Psychology*, **2** (3) 3–22.

Hakim, C. (1987) *Research Design: Strategies and Choices in the Design of Social Research*, George Allen & Unwin, London.

Hammersley, M. and Atkinson, P. (1983) *Ethnography: Principles in Practice*, Tavistock, London.

Hannah, K., Gullemin, F. and Conklin, D.N. (1986) *Nursing Uses of Computers and Information Science*; North Holland, Amsterdam.

Harris, R.B. and Hyman, R.B. (1984) 'Clean vs. sterile: tracheotomy care and level of pulmonary infection', *Nursing Research*, **33** (2) 80–5.

Hastings, E.H. and Hastings, P.K. (eds) (1980) *Index to International Public Opinion 1978–1979*, Greenwood Press, Westport, Connecticut.

Henshaw. A. and Schepp, K. (1984) 'Problems in doing nursing research: how to recognise garbage when you see it!', *Western Journal of Nursing*, **6**, 126–30.

Heyman, R., Shaw, M.P., and Harding, J. (1983) 'A personal construct theory approach to socialization of nursing trainees in two British general hospitals', *Journal of Advanced Nursing*, **8**, 59–67.

Hoinville, G., Jowell, R. and associates (1978) *Survey Research Practice*, Heinemann, London.

Jocobson, S.F. (1983) 'Stresses and coping strategies of neonatal intensive care unit nurses', *Research in Nursing and Health*, **6**, 33–40.

Jacobson, S.F. (1984) 'A semantic differential for external comparison of conceptual nursing models', *Advances in Nursing Science*, **6**, 58–70.

Jick, T.D. (1983) 'Mixing qualitative and quantitative methods: triangulation in action' in J. Van Maanen (ed.) *Qualitative Methodology*, Sage, Beverly Hills, California, pp. 135–48.

Kelly, G. (1963) *A Theory of Personality: The Psychology of Personal Constructs*, Norton, New York.

Kerlinger, F.N. (1986) *Foundation of Behavioral Research*, 3rd edn, CBS, New York.

Kirk, J. and Miller, M.L. (1986) *Reliability and Validity in Qualitative Research*, Sage, London.

Knaak, P. (1984) 'Phenomenological research', *Western Journal of Nursing Research* **6**, 107–14.

Knafl, K.A. and Howard, K.J. (1984) 'Interpreting and reporting qualitative research', *Research in Nursing and Health*, **7**, 17–24.

Kogan, M. and Henkely, M. (1983) *Government and Research: The Rothschild Experiment in a Government Department*, Heinemann, London.

Kovacs, A.R. (1985) *The Research Process: Essentials of Skill Development*, F.A. Davis, Philadelphia.

Krampitz, S.D. and Pavlovich, N. (1981) *Readings for Nursing Research*, C.V. Mosby, St Louis.

Krippendorff, K. (1980) *Content Analysis: An Introduction to Its Methodology*, Sage, Beverly Hills, California.

Kvale, S. (1983) 'The qualitative research interview: a phenomenological and hermeneutical mode of understanding', *Journal of Phenomenological Psychology*, *14* (2) 171–96.

Kvale, S. (1987) 'Interpretation of the qualitative research interview', in F.J. van Zuuren, F. Wertz, and B. Mook (eds) *Advances in Qualitative Psychology*, Swets & Zeitlinger BV, Lisse, pp. 25–40.

Leininger, M.M. (ed.) (1985) *Qualitative Research Methods in Nursing*, Grune & Stratton, New York.

Macleod Clark, J. and Hockey, L. (1979) *Research for Nursing: A Guide for the Enquiring Nurse'* H.M. & M., London.

Manis, J.G. and Meltzer, B.N. (1978) *Symbolic Interaction*, Allyn & Bacon, Boston, Massachusetts.

Marsh, C. (1982) *The Survey Method*, George Allen & Unwin, London.

Marshall, L.A. and Rowland, F. (1983) *A Guide to Learning Independently*, Open University Press, Milton Keynes.

Martin, P.Y. and Turner, B.A. (1986) 'Grounded Theory and Organisational Research', *Journal of Applied Behavioural Science*, **22**, 141–58.

Mishel, M.H. (1981) 'The measurement of uncertainty in illness', *Nursing Research*, **30**, 258–63.

Morrison, P. (1990) 'An example of the use of repertory grid technique in assessing nurses' self-perceptions of caring', *Nurse Education Today*, **10**, 253–9.

Mostyn, B. (1985) 'The content analysis of qualitative research data: a dynamic approach' in M. Brenner, J. Brown, and D. Canter (eds) *The Research Interview: Uses and Approaches*, Academic Press, London, pp. 115–45.

Moyser, G. and Wagstaffe, M. (eds) (1987) *Research Methods for Elite Studies*, Allen & Unwin, London.

Munhall, P.L. and Oiler, C.J. (1986) *Nursing Research: A Qualitative Perspective*, Appleton-Century-Crofts, Connecticut.

Notter, L.E. (1979) *Essentials of Nursing Research*, 2nd edn, Tavistock, London.

Oiler, C. (1982) 'The Phenomenological Approach in Nursing Research', *Nursing Research*, **31**, 178–81.

Oppenheim, A.N. (1992) *Questionnaire Design, Intertaining and Attitude Measurement*, 3rd edn. Pinter, London.

Osgood, C.E., Suci, G.J. and Tannenbaum, P.H. (1957) *The Measurement of Meaning*, University of Illinois Press, Urbana.

Paradoo, K. and Reid, N. (1988) 'Research skills number 1, getting started:

the language of research', *Nursing Times*, **84** (39) 67–70.

Polgar, S. and Thomas, S.A. (1991) *Introduction to Research in the Health Sciences*, 2nd edn, Churchill Livingstone, Melbourne.

Pollock, L.C. (1987) 'Community Psychiatric Nursing Explained: An Analysis of the Views of Patients, Carers and Nurses', unpublished PhD thesis, University of Edinburgh.

Popper, K.R. (1959) *The Logic of Scientific Method*, Hutchinson, London.

Reid, N. (1993) *Health Care Research by Degrees*, Blackwell, Oxford.

Research in British Universities, Polytechnics and Colleges, British Library, London.

Roberts, H. (ed.) (1981) *Doing Feminist Research*, Routledge & Kegan Paul, London.

Rowntree, D. (1981) *Statistics without Tears*, Penguin, London.

Schlenker, B.R. (1980) *Impression Management: The Self-Concept, Social Identity, and Interpersonal Relations*, Belmont, California, Brooks/Cole.

Shipman, M. (1981) *The Limitations of Social Research*, 2nd edn, Longmans, London.

Shotter, J. (1975) *Images of Man in Psychological Research*, Methuen, London.

Shye, S. (ed.) (1978) *Theory Construction and Data Analysis in the Behavioral Sciences*, Jossey-Bass, San Francisco.

Silverman, D. (1985) *Qualitative Methodology in Sociology*, Gower, Aldershot.

Spilker, B. (1984) *A Guide to Clinical Studies and Developing Protocols*, Raven Press, New York.

Spindler, G. (ed.) (1982) *Doing the Ethnography of Schooling: Educational Anthropology in Action*, Holt, Rinehart & Winston, New York.

Spradley, J.A. (1980) *Participant Observation*, Holt, Rinehart & Winston, New York.

Sudman, S. and Bradburn, N.M. (1982) *Asking Questions: A Practical Guide to Questionnaire Design*, Jossey Bass, San Francisco.

Sudman, S. and Lannom, L.B. (1980) *Health Care Surveys Using Diaries*, NCHSR Research Report 80–4, National Center for Health Services Research, Hyattsville, Maryland.

Swanson, J.M. and Chenitz, W.C. (1982) 'Why qualitative research in nursing?' *Nursing Outlook*, **30**, 241–5.

Sweeney, M.A. (1985) *The Nurse's Guide to Computers*, Macmillan, New York.

Taylor, S.J. and Bogdan, R. (1984) *Introduction to Qualitative Research Methods: The Search for Meanings*, 2nd edn, Wiley, New York.

Tornquist, E.M. (1986) *From Proposal to Publication: An Informal Guide to Writing About Nursing Research*, Addison Wesley, Menlo Park, New York.

Turabian, K.L. (1973) *A Manual for Writers of Term Papers, Theses and Dissertations*, 4th edn, University of Chicago Press, Chicago.

Turner, B.A. (1981) 'Some practical aspects of qualitative data analysis:

one way of organising some of the cognitive processes associated with the generation of grounded theory', *Quality and Quantity*, **15**, 225–47.

United Nations Statistical Year Book, United Nations, New York. Published annually.

United States Library of Congress: The National Union Catalogue, Boston, Massachusetts.

Van Maanen, J. (1983) *Qualitative Methodology*, Sage, Beverly Hills, California.

Van Zuuren, F.J., Wertz, F., and Mook, B. (eds) (1987) *Advances in Qualitative Psychology: Themes and Variations*, Swetz & Zeitlinger BV Lisse.

Viney, L.L. (1988) 'A PCP analysis of data collection in the social sciences', in F. Fransella and L. Thomas (eds) *Experimenting With Personal Construct Psychology*, Routledge & Kegan Paul, London, pp. 369–80.

Walsh, R. (ed.) (1985) *A Bibliography of Nursing Literature, Vol. 3*, Library Association Publishing, London.

Waltz, C.F. and Bausell, R.B. (1981) *Nursing Research: Design, Statistics and Computer Analysis*, F.A. Davis Philadelphia.

Waltz, C.F., Strickland, O.L. and Lenz, E.R. (1984) *Measurement in Nursing Research*, F.A. Davis, Philadelphia.

Watson, J. (1985) *Nursing: Human Science and Human Care: A Theory of Nursing*, Appleton-Century-Crofts, Connecticut.

Wattley, L.A. and Muller, D (1984) *Investigating Psychology: A Practical Approach for Nursing*, Harper & Row, London.

Wax, R. (1971) *Doing Fieldwork: Warnings and Advice*, University of Chicago Press, Chicago.

Wenger, G.C. (ed.) (1987) *The Research Relationship*, Allen & Unwin, London.

White, J.H. (1984) 'The relationship of clinical practice and research', *Journal of Advanced Nursing*, **9**, 181–7.

Whyte, W.F. (1955) *Street Corner Society*, 2nd edn, University of Chicago Press, Chicago.

Wilkinson, D. (1982) 'The effects of brief psychiatric training on the attitudes of general nursing students to psychiatric patients', *Journal of Advanced Nursing*, **7**, 239–53.

Wilson, H.S. (1985) *Research in Nursing*, Addison Wesley, Menlo Park, New York.

Winstead-Fry, P. (ed.) (1986) *Case Studies in Nursing Theory*, National League for Nursing, New York.

Woods, N.F. (1988) *Nursing Research: A Learning Resource*, Mosby, St Louis.

Yin, R. (1984) *Case Study Research: Design and Method*, Applied Social Research Series no. 5, Sage, Beverly Hills, California.

Zelditch, M. Jr (1969) 'Some methodological problems of field studies', in B.J. McCall and J.L. Simmons (eds) *Issues in Participant Observation: A Text and Reader*; Addison-Wesley, Menlo Park, California.

Index

179